The Return of Epidemics

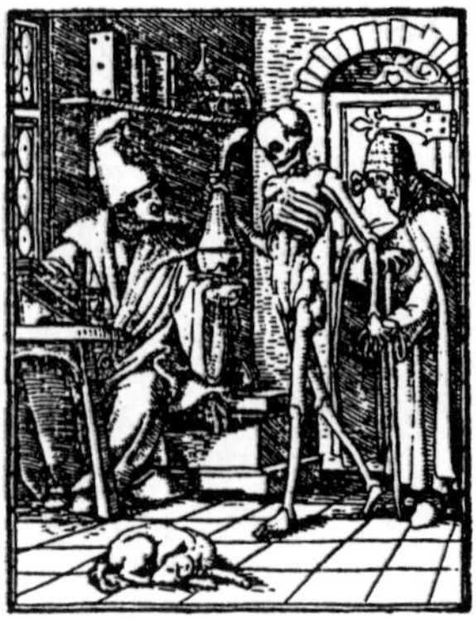

The History of Medicine in Context

Series Editors: Andrew Cunningham and Ole Peter Grell,
Department of History and Philosophy of Science,
University of Cambridge

Titles in this series include:

Medicine from the Black Death to the French Disease
edited by Roger French, Jon Arrizabalaga,
Andrew Cunningham and Luis García-Ballester

Faith, Medical Alchemy and Natural Philosophy:
Johann Moriaen, Reformed Intelligencer, and the Hartlib Circle
John T. Young

The Making of the Dentiste, c. *1650–1760*
Roger King

'The Battle for Health': A Political History of the
Socialist Medical Association, 1930–51
John Stewart

Medicine and Charity in Georgian Bath:
A Social History of the General Infirmary, c. *1739–1830*
Anne Borsay

The Nurse Apprentice, 1860–1977
Ann Bradshaw

The Return of Epidemics

Health and Society in Peru during the Twentieth Century

MARCOS CUETO

Ashgate

Aldershot • Burlington USA • Singapore • Sydney

Published by
Ashgate Publishing Limited
Gower House
Croft Road
Aldershot
Hants GU11 3HR
England

Ashgate Publishing Company
131 Main Street
Burlington
Vermont 05401–5600
USA

Ashgate website: http://www.ashgate.com

British Library Cataloguing in Publication Data

Cueto, Marcos.
The Return of Epidemics: Health and Society in Peru during the Twentieth Century.
(The History of Medicine in Context)
1. Epidemics—Peru—History—20th century. 2. Public health—Peru—History—20th century. 3. Medical policy—Peru—History—20th century. 4. Social medicine—Peru—History—20th century.
I. Title.
306.4'61'0985'0904

Library of Congress Cataloging-in-Publication Data

Cueto, Marcos.
The return of epidemics: health and society in Peru during the twentieth century/Marcos Cueto.
p. cm. (The History of Medicine in Context)
Includes bibliographical references and index.
ISBN 0–7546–0314–8 (alk. paper)
1. Epidemics—Peru—History—20th century. 2. Social medicine—Peru—History—20th century. I. Title. II. Series.
RA650.55.P5.C843 2001
614.4'985'0904—dc21 00–48496

ISBN 0 7546 0314 8

This book is printed on acid free paper
Typeset in Times by N²productions
Printed and bound by Athenaeum Press, Ltd., Gateshead, Tyne & Wear.

Contents

Acknowledgements

As is the case for many other books this one appears thanks to the support of several people and institutions. Among the latter are the Social Science Research Council, the John Simon Guggenheim Memorial Foundation, the Rockefeller Archive Center, the Program in Science, Technology and Society of the Massachusetts Institute of Technology, the Ministry of Foreign Relations of Spain, the Wellcome Trust, the Pan American Health Organization, the National Library of Medicine, the Consejo Latinoamericano de Ciencias Sociales, the Instituto de Estudios Peruanos, the Universidad Peruana Cayetano Heredia and the Peruvian Council of Science and Technology. These institutions provided me with grants and/or logistic support that made my research possible. A special mention has to be made to the Latin American Studies Association that declared a Spanish version of this work published by the Instituto de Estudios Peruanos a co-winner of the *Premio Iberoamericano* for 1998.

I am also very grateful to the libraries, archives and families holding papers of individuals, mentioned in the bibliography, for giving me access to their valuable materials. My thanks to the interviewees who provided data, insight and documents. I am also grateful to the young Peruvian historians who worked as my research assistants in different stages of my study: Jorge Lossio, César Salas, Jorge Blanco and the late Mario Marcone. Several friends and colleagues offered me advice and encouragement during my research: my thanks are due to Nancy Leys Stepan, Darwin Stapleton, Herbert S. Klein, Jon Arrizabalaga, Anne Emanuelle Birn, Jaime Benchimol, Julyan Peard, Thomas Glick, Jorge Cañizares, Stuart McCook, Ronald Numbers, Diego Armus, Diana Obregón, Uriel García, Guenther Risse, Emilio Quevedo, Paul Wendling, Carlos Contreras, Alfonso Quiroz, Rafael Varón, Roger Guerra-García, Antonio Lafuente and the late Eduardo Estrella.

I am especially grateful to Javier Flores, who did a remarkable job in preparing the English version of the manuscript. I am certain that the questions, criticism and suggestions of the students and colleagues of Cayetano Heredia inspired and polished my research.

My special thanks to Andrew Cunningham and Ole Peter Grell, the series editors of 'The History of Medicine in Context', and to Caroline Cornish and Rachel Lynch at Ashgate who assisted me with care, efficiency and expert advice in the preparation of the book.

The courtesy of the editors of *The Hispanic American Historical Review* and *The Bulletin of the History of Medicine* allows me to use the materials (now appearing in chapters two and three) that were originally published in these journals in the volumes of 1992 and 1991 respectively.

Finally, I owe my family – Cecilia, Vicente, Alejandra and Rodrigo – a great debt of thanks. This book is dedicated to them.

Marcos Cueto

Abbreviations

ACCT	Archivo de la Cámara de Comercio de Trujillo, Trujillo
ADA	Archivo Departamental de Ayacucho, Ayacucho
ADCa	Archivo Departamental de Cajamarca, Cajamarca
ADCu	Archivo Departamental del Cuzco, Cuzco
ADLa	Archivo Departamental de Lambayeque, Chiclayo
ADP	Archivo Departamental de Piura, Piura
ADPu	Archivo Departamental de Puno, Puno
AGHUB	Archivo General e Histórico de la Universidad de Barcelona, Barcelona
AGN	Archivo General de la Nación, Lima
AHBMC	Archivo Histórico de la Biblioteca Municipal del Cuzco, Cuzco
AID	Agencia Internacional de Desarrollo (International Development Agency)
AIDS	acquired immune deficiency syndrome
AMPa	Archivo Municipal de Paita, Piura
AMPi	Archivo Municipal de Piura, Piura
APRA	Alianza Popular Revolucionaria Americana (Popular Revolutionary American Alliance)
BMP	Biblioteca Municipal de Piura, Piura
BN	Oficina de Investigaciones Bibliográficas y Fondos Especiales de la Biblioteca Nacional, Lima
DC	*Diario de Chimbote*, Chimbote
DDT	dichlorodiphenyltrichloroethane
DISABAR	Division of Basic Rural Environmental Sanitation
EC	*El Comercio*, Lima
ED	*El Deber*, Piura
EGP	*El Grito del Pueblo*, Ferreñafe
EPA	Environmental Protection Agency
ES(P)	*El Sol*, Piura
ES(C)	*El Sol*, Cuzco
ET	*El Tiempo*, Chiclayo
ET(P)	*El Tiempo*, Piura
K	*Kanatari*, Iquitos
LI(C)	*La Industria*, Chiclayo
LI(P)	*La Industria*, Piura
LI(T)	*La Industria*, Trujillo
LR	*La Reforma*, Trujillo
NA	National Archives, Washington, DC
O	*Oiga*, Lima

PAHO	Pan American Health Organization
PMNB-A	Papeles de Manuel Núñez Butrón, Arequipa
PMNB-L	Papeles de Manuel Núñez Butrón, Lima
RAC	Rockefeller Archive Center, New York
RF	Rockefeller Foundation
RFA	Rockefeller Foundation Archive
RS	*Runa Soncco*, Juliaca
RSD	*Resumen Semanal, Desco*, Lima
S	*Satélite*, Trujillo
SCISP	Servicio Cooperativo Interamericano de Salud Pública
SENAPA	National Water Supply and Sewage Service
UNICEF	United Nations Children's Fund
UROs	Oral Rehydration Units

Introduction

Epidemics are no longer distant catastrophes but are a tragic reality in poor and underdeveloped countries.[1] This is related to the frustration of the dream that developed at the turn of twentieth century of conquering the infectious diseases, to the rise of new pathologies like acquired immune deficiency syndrome (AIDS) and the Ebola virus, and to a redefinition of the term to include any disease that intensively attacks a group by surprise. Some historians have cogently argued that epidemics are the hidden and true factor in history that explains the outcome of several events.[2] For instance, that Greek civilization actually declined due to malaria, that the Middle Ages ended because of the Black Death or that the Incas were defeated by the smallpox and measles which came from the Old World.[3] Besides, epidemics have fascinated historians for other reasons too.

The study of epidemics enabled the study of the ecological foundations of collective diseases, and revealed areas of the social fabric which do not appear clearly in everyday life.[4] An epidemic heightens the relation between economic systems and living conditions; illuminates little known areas of the *mentalités*, ideologies and religious beliefs, and illustrates efforts and inadequacies in the preservation of public health.[5] Epidemics sometimes are a stimulus for the expansion of the State's authority into social areas which, like health, were not always its responsibility, and have sometimes served like a magnifying glass for the study of the fears, prejudices, rules and stereotypes regarding the sick, the human body, gender, ethnic groups and the poor.[6] The variety of perceptions, practices and testimonies which come to the surface during an epidemic remind us that a disease is not just a simple biological fact of concern only to physicians.

Past epidemics have been of interest to a series of studies of Africa and India which are part of one of the most dynamic areas of social history: the history of medicine in the colonies or in Third World countries. These studies have shown that public health was sometimes a tool for the increase of productivity in areas under economic exploitation, for the protection of the health of colonizers, for the development of stereotypes announcing the inferiority of the natives and for the diffusion of the presumed superiority of western culture, which included a more rational, efficient and humanitarian medicine.[7] Some of the critiques made against this literature are that it pays scant attention to the natural history of disease, and concentrates on the perceptions western doctors have of the underdeveloped parts of the world, without giving due attention to the popular perception of disease or the patterns of the responses that ordinary people give to sanitary policies.

Save for some demographic studies of the colonial period, the history of epidemics is a new area of study in Peruvian and Latin American historiography.[8] Traditional Peruvian historians of medicine, like Hermilio Valdizán and Juan B. Lastres, undertook a remarkable work some decades ago on popular perceptions of medicine, and then concentrated on reconstructing the institutional development of western medicine. Unfortunately, their work was only sparingly followed. One of the goals of this book is to help Peruvian and Latin American history enlarge its research agenda to include health and disease as important areas of the past for an understanding of the living conditions of the people, of popular conceptions of well-being and physical and mental breakdown, of the consolidation of the State's authority and of the dynamics of social movements.

The aim of this study is to contribute to the national and international history of epidemics and medicine through the study of the causes, the impact and the responses given to several diseases that attacked various parts of Peru during the twentieth century.[9] One thing that distinguishes this study is that it does not concentrate on just one type of ailment but on several diseases that plagued the Peruvian people, in an attempt to establish recurring individual, social and governmental response patterns. One of the objectives of this study is to reconcile the natural and social history of disease by giving due attention both to those factors that explain the ecology of epidemics in Peru, as well as to social reactions to disease.

Epidemics were due mainly to poverty and also to the lack of an adequate sanitary infrastructure. They usually began with an unexpected outbreak which was identified after some initial confusion. It was only when the disease gained strength that emergency measures were taken, which sometimes included establishing organizations that ended up forming part of the State. There were also popular reactions like flight from affected areas, blaming the contagion on marginal groups or on groups perceived as alien, the resistance shown to authoritarian sanitary methods, and the later toning down both of the epidemic and the sanitary measures. In each epidemic I study three aspects: its impact, with a brief discussion of the biological and ecological factors that cause it, the techniques and policies applied to fight it and the social responses.

The study of sanitary policies describes the institutional development of health organizations, the development of control and eradication campaigns by Peruvian and international institutions, the use of vaccines, serums or disinfection and fumigation techniques, and the practices of physicians, quacks and Indian healers. The study of the social responses includes the attitudes shown by regional authorities, the Church, merchants, physicians and popular sectors in the face of measures such as the suspension of trade and communications through the closing down of ports, the unemployment caused by quarantines, the incineration of dwellings, the segregation of the sick and the introduction of sanitary techniques that affected customs. Since the definition of each disease varies for each cultural group that faces it and changes over time, I have tried not to appraise the historical actors in relation to their knowledge or ignorance of contemporary scientific knowledge on diseases.[10]

The first chapter presents the bubonic plague that affected Peru's major coastal cities in 1903–30. This epidemic showed the hazardous conditions of urban life, the overlapping division of labour between sanitary organizations and a propensity to blame the disease on subaltern groups like the Chinese immigrants. In this first epidemic there were physicians who bravely looked after the sick in adverse conditions, and faced the quandary health workers would long face – should they treat people, or promote long-term measures like environmental sanitation and the organization of stable sanitary institutions? The establishment in 1903 of the Bureau of Public Health, the first national health agency, shows that the early twentieth-century health workers managed to make some good use of the campaign against the plague.

The second chapter describes the yellow fever epidemic of 1919–22 that struck major north coast harbours and sugar-producing localities, and which was controlled thanks to the intervention of the Rockefeller Foundation. In this campaign, sanitary measures were applied in an authoritarian fashion, with great confidence in the intrinsic power of technological resources, little emphasis on community educational programmes, and an idea that would prove lasting – that the people were one of the major obstacles that had to be overcome in the struggle against epidemics.

The third chapter focuses on the efforts made to fight epidemic typhus and smallpox in the Andes, and to combine sanitation with a regional cultural movement known as indigenism. The leading characters in this story were the physician Manuel Núñez Butrón and some rural sanitary brigades that worked in Puno in the 1930s. This case illustrates a successful attempt at self-help and collaboration with the natural leaders of the communities, and emphasizes the capability of the people to give creative and efficient responses in the face of adversity.

The fourth chapter studies the successive campaigns for the control and eradication of malaria, an endemic disease in the coastlands and the tropical forest throughout the twentieth century. Special attention is given to the epidemic that struck Quillabamba in 1932, in the tropical forest of Cuzco. This violent epidemic revealed the precarious condition of the migrant population, the unstable nature of the colonization of the tropical forest and the reluctance of the *hacendados* to prepare a sanitary infrastructure. The chapter emphasizes the significance that differential disease patterns had according to the traditional geographical division of Peru into coast, highlands and tropical forest.

The study of the environmental barriers presented by these patterns and their turning point in the 1960s, allows for a better understanding of the encounter and opposition of different cultural groups. For example, the control of malaria was one of the major stimuli for migration from the highlands to the coast from 1950 to 1970. Up to then, the disease had attacked highland migrants who worked seasonally on the coast in preference to other groups. These workers often resisted migrating to the coast because of the overexploitation they were subject to, and because of diseases like malaria. A remarkable control of the disease was attained since the 1950s by the use of insecticides such as dichlorodiphenyltrichloroethane (DDT), and this stimulated migration from the highlands to the coast and the tropical forest. This finding does not seek to diminish the significance which the agrarian crisis, urbanization and industrialization all had on the migratory process, but rather to add an element missing in social history – the real and perceived impact of a disease. This same chapter discusses the aborted eradication of malaria which took place in the 1950s. Failure set the stage for a time when less importance would be given to public health.

The fifth chapter examines the 1991 cholera epidemic which caused over 322 000 casualties, and dealt a blow to the export of fish, the food trade and tourism, while rapidly becoming a symbol of the general crisis that then prevailed in Peru. The major legacy of this epidemic was that it consolidated a trend that blamed the disease on its victims, reinforced the social exclusion of the poor, downplayed the significance of environmental sanitation and considered public health as an individual and family matter, and not as one of the duties of the State.

The title of this book is an allusion to the feedback between poverty and disease. Every given number of years, poor countries like Peru once again come face to face with an epidemic that usually provokes authoritarian, controllist and insufficient responses. It is worth emphasizing, as the European nineteenth-century health workers did, that poverty produces disease, but diseases also produce poverty which is reflected in unemployment and the inability to come to grips with life and death.

This book seeks to be relevant in contemporary terms. The study of epidemics can contribute to a modern conceptualization of Peru and its health and social challenges, that is, a reflection with a long-term approach focused on the gap between social problems and the resources available to solve them, the limitations of individual efforts in the struggle against adversity, the relationship between ethnic fragmentation and authoritarian and discontinuous social policies, the real and imagined difficulties different human groups have had to endure together and the recurrence of temporal solutions as a response to crises.

At the beginning of the twenty-first century, Peruvians are experiencing a major change in their sanitary services, the return of several epidemics which in the recent past had seemed to be controlled, and the threat that new epidemics will be unleashed. The writer hopes this study will suggest that the future can, in fact, be different and better.

Notes

1. See Elizabeth Fee and Daniel Fox (eds), *AIDS: The Burdens of History*, University of California Press, Berkeley, 1990; Charles Rosenberg, *Explaining Epidemics and Other Studies in the History of Medicine*, Cambridge University Press, Cambridge, 1992; Laurie Garrett, *The Coming Plague, Newly Emerging Diseases in a World Out of Balance*, Penguin Books, New York, 1995.
2. William McNeill, *Plagues and Peoples*, Double Day, New York, 1976; Alfred Crosby, *The Columbian Exchange: Biological and Cultural Consequences of 1492*, Greenwood Press, Westport, CT, 1972.
3. See Guenter B. Risse, 'Epidemics Before Aids: A New Research Program', in Victoria Harden and Guenter B. Risse (eds), *Aids and the Historian*, National Institute of Health, Washington, DC, 1991, pp. 2–12, for the various usages of epidemics among physicians, historians and writers.
4. Charles Rosenberg, *The Cholera Years: The United States in 1832, 1849, and 1866*, University of Chicago Press, Chicago, 1962; Richard Evans, *Death in Hamburg, Society and Politics in the Cholera Years, 1830–1910*, Penguin Books, London, 1987; Paul Slack, *The Impact of Plague in Tudor and Stuart England*, Oxford University Press, Oxford, 1990; Terence Ranger and Paul Slack, *Epidemics and Ideas, Essays on the History of Pestilence*, Cambridge University Press, Cambridge, 1992.
5. Michael Durey, *The Return of the Plague, British Society and the Cholera, 1831–1832*, Gill and Macmillan Humanities Press, Dublin, 1979; Carlos Cipolla, *Fighting the Plague in Seventeenth-Century Italy*, University of Wisconsin Press, Madison, WI, 1981.
6. François Delaporte, *Disease and Civilization, the Cholera in Paris, 1832*, Massachusetts Institute of Technology, Cambridge, MA, 1986.
7. Some of the most recent studies are David Arnold, *Colonizing the Body, State Medicine and Epidemic Disease in Nineteenth Century India*, University of California Press, Berkeley, CA, 1993; Mark Harrison, *Public Health in British India, Anglo-Indian Preventive Medicine, 1859–1914*, Cambridge University Press, Cambridge, 1994. For Latin America, see Renán Silva, *Las epidemias de la viruela de 1782 y 1802 en la Nueva Granada*, Universidad del Valle, Cali, 1992; Donald Cooper, *Epidemic Disease in Mexico City, 1761–1813: An Administrative, Social and Medical Study*, University of Texas Press, Austin, TX, 1965.
8. Noble David Cook, *Demographic Collapse: Indian Peru, 1520–1620*, Cambridge University Press, Cambridge, 1981; Henry Dobyns, 'An Outline of Andean Epidemic History to 1720', *Bulletin of the History of Medicine*, **37**, 1963, pp. 493–515; José Toribio Polo, *Apuntes sobre las epidemias en el Perú*, Federico Barrionuevo, Lima, 1913, pp. 50–109.
9. See 'Introduction' to Marcos Cueto (ed.), *Missionaries of Science: The Rockefeller Foundation and Latin America*, Indiana University Press, Bloomington, IN, 1994, p. ix.
10. For a discussion of the changing definition of disease, see Andrew Cunningham, 'Transforming Plague: The Laboratory and the Identity of Infectious Disease', in Andrew Cunningham and Perry Williams (eds), *The Laboratory Revolution in Medicine*, Cambridge University Press, Cambridge, 1992, p. 209.

CHAPTER ONE

The Stigma of Bubonic Plague in Early Twentieth-Century Peru

The port of Callao, 1st May 1903.

While dressing the body of her son Pedro for the burial, Mrs Figueroa noticed an abnormal swelling on the neck of the corpse. Her discovery went unheeded for the next days, until ten of the seventy men who worked in the mill with Pedro Figueroa fell seriously ill with an unknown disease that parched their tongue, swelled their eyes, gave them severe headaches, plunged them into fever and caused buboes the size of a pigeon's egg on their necks, the groins, and armpits. Perhaps some then reflected that there might be a connection between their suffering, the death of Pedro, and the stench from the dead rats in the mill.[1]

This was one of the first accounts in Peru of a terrible epidemic of bubonic plague, a disease that is transmitted by the bite of fleas – usually the *Xenopsylla cheopis* – from rats infected with the *Yersinia pestis* bacterium. An outbreak among humans is preceded by an epizooty of rodents, that is, the death of the infected rats, and causes death in untreated patients within two months of infection.[2] The plague extended to Lima and the major ports of Peru in 1903–05, and shortly thereafter became a characteristic trait of all coastal departments, and of some in the highlands. The serious inadequacies of urban life came to light in the years the disease was endemic (1903–30), while the sanitation policies which were advocated were distinguished by palliative measures, and various social and individual responses that were related to fear, cultural differences and economic interests.

Rats and the plague

In the early twentieth century, the environment in Lima and other coastal areas was ideal for rats and mice. These rodents could easily spread due to the excessive population, overcrowded living conditions, rickety dwellings, piles of refuse and unhygienic habits. These customs included urinating and defecating in the streets, and casting out any piece of rubbish, relying on the appetite of buzzards, dogs, donkeys and other animals that wandered about in the streets. A partial solution to this problem was removing refuse in wagons to the garbage dumps, which appeared in the late colonial period as a way of concentrating refuse in marginal urban areas. For instance, a great part of the

60 tons of refuse that were produced daily in Lima around 1903, were taken to the dumps located on the banks of the Rímac River. By then these dumps were already within the urban perimeter. Pigs fed on swill in the dump by the Tajamar, and there was a slaughterhouse near another dump in Monserrat.[3] The lack of an efficient refuse-disposal system was compounded by the poor condition of the sewers. Notwithstanding the various attempts made to establish closed sewers since the mid-nineteenth century, most urban areas had open sewers running through the streets. Major cities like Lima had a closed but precarious sewage system, and houses had shallow silos which were magnificent breeding grounds for rats.[4]

In general, houses were unhygienic and not enough of them were available. Although Lima expanded its urban perimeter by more than a kilometre between 1896 and 1904, the living and sanitary services were not those needed by a population that had rapidly grown from 100 194 inhabitants in 1896, to 139 289 in 1903.[5] Most homes had hollow walls, wide spaces between the boarded floor and the ground, mud bricks on the ground floor, and walls of wattle and daub on the upper storey, that is, suitable living conditions for rats. According to a contemporary report, not even the best houses in Lima were made of concrete (which would have prevented the entry of rats).[6] There were plenty of ideal living conditions for the rodents at the other end of the social scale. Among the poorest coastal populations, dwellings consisted of a small elevated room made of mud or reeds, markets were improvised on river banks from whence they polluted the waters and the environment, and streets were narrow and winding and were not paved.

Inefficient refuse-disposal systems, overcrowded dwellings, and untended storehouses of food and cereals which attracted rats were prevalent in several coastal areas. In the port of Mollendo, the most important outlet for merchandise in southern Peru, wooden houses were built over an inclined plane. Their base formed an empty space, known as a *sucucho*, where refuse was placed and rodents lived.[7] On the opposite extreme, Paita, the port of entry to the north, was composed of reed huts raised over dirt streets, and the wooden warehouses of the shipping and retail companies. According to a local physician, '[t]he nature of the buildings ... is ideal for housing the germ of the pest indefinitely. Few, very few are the houses that can be ... disinfected'.[8]

Another side to the housing problem of the major cities was overcrowding. In Lima, for example, the high ceilings and big rooms of the old mansions were divided with wooden partitions to form several floors of small dwellings. The object of these subdivisions was to pack in the highest possible number of tenants. These mansions housed several destitute families. A physician vividly described the inside of one of these dwellings:

> On reaching the second storey we found it made up of narrow passageways ... the so-called ... apartments are on each side, as they only have a room ... 2 to 3 metres long, to which light and air enter through a small door, on

> top of which is a small window which is often covered by canvas, and so the total darkness inside can be imagined ... the high humidity makes each room a focus of contagion, wherein live ... from 2 to 6 individuals and more.[9]

Another form of overcrowded housing developed in downtown Lima: the *callejones*. These were one-storey dwellings with a long corridor running through them, with the apartments – usually no more than one room – opening at each side. *Callejones* usually had no sanitation, and their water supply was just a fountain in the corridor, at the end facing the main doorway. In these urban dwellings, poor families, dirt and, of course, rats, found refuge. The following statement from a newspaper was most likely not an isolated case: 'Huge, almost domesticated rats live there, in gentle intimacy with the neighbourhood's children.'[10]

The epidemic made physicians emphasize the precarious living conditions. For instance, in late 1904 the type of dwelling from whence came the 386 plague cases interned in the isolation hospital, or lazaretto, was appraised, and it showed that most (126) were *callejones*.[11] The physician Rómulo Eyzaguirre estimated the percentage of people living in less than one room in each of the five sectors into which Lima was divided. The study gave a high overcrowding rate that varied between 55 per cent in the second sector (the lowest one) and 78 per cent in the fifth one (the highest). Eyzaguirre also related the percentage of overcrowding with race and found that the most overcrowded sector corresponded mostly to Indian and mestizo populations (52 per cent in the fifth sector). This, plus the fact that the fifth sector beside the Rímac River was distinguished by having poor families and the three major dumps in the city, explains why this sector had the highest number of patients in the lazaretto (111 out of a total of 386.)[12]

The growth of international trade in the early twentieth century worsened the conditions which abetted the proliferation of rodents, as it increased contacts between Peruvian ports and ships from areas where the plague was endemic. In Peru, the plague was assumed to have arrived from Bangkok – the focus of the plague pandemic that swept throughout the world from 1894 onwards – with the *Serapis*, which berthed in Callao in late December 1902 with over 10 000 sacks of rice for the Milne mill.[13] The increase in the number of voyages, passengers, merchandise and rats moving from one Peruvian port to the other, placed healthy populations in contact with sick ones. The intensification of marine trade stimulated the unplanned growth of cities and ports. The urbanization of the country was always faster than the supply of sanitation facilities, a pattern that would last throughout the twentieth century.

The development of the plague in the major coastal cities appears in Table 1.1, which indicates that the epidemics came in irregular waves, and tended to reach their low point wherever the first outbreak was severe. The most common form of the plague was the bubonic plague, less contagious and harder to

Table 1.1 Cases of bubonic plague on the north coast of Peru, 1903–30

Years	Paita	Chiclayo	Pacasmayo	Trujillo	Lima	Total*
1903–05	254	282	377	106	533	1 873
1906–10	321	542	433	1 729	783	4 300
1911–15	45	444	367	978	611	3 649
1916–20	236	132	295	814	492	3 017
1921–25	169	230	140	422	699	3 448
1926–30	16	133	270	244	322	1 556
Total	1 041	1 763	1 882	4 293	3 440	17 843

* Includes other locations on the north coast.

Source: C.R. Eskey, 'Epidemiological Study of Plague in Peru, 1931' R.G. 90, United States Public Health Service, Foreign Governments, 'Peru', File 0425, Box 37, National Archives, Washington, DC.

acquire than the other two kinds (pneumonic and septicemic).[14] The disease reached its first maximum point in 1908 with 1691 cases, and its second one with 1200 cases in 1926, after some torrential rains.[15] The rains flooded the lairs of the rodents, thus abetting the invasion of houses by rats. Despite its spectacular nature, the plague never caused a higher death rate than other infectious diseases like tuberculosis.

By 1910 the plague changed from a disease centred around ports, to another with a rural niche, in country rats which perhaps in turn infected the guinea pigs by moving to houses in search of shelter and food. The rats went to the warehouses in the attic – a wooden floor close to the roof – where maize, cereal and other crops were stored. The fleas fell directly to the floor once the rodents died in these attics, and found a new source of food and objects for infection in human beings.

The plague was particularly severe on the north coast during the first two decades of this century. Towards the end of the second decade, it spread with intensity to low-altitude Andean areas like the highlands of the coastal departments of Piura and Lambayeque and in the highland department of Cajamarca. This was due to the transportation of infected lice in the merchandise carried by the muleteers engaged in commercial transport between the coast and the highlands.[16] Highland communities also became reinfected through contact with endemic centres on the coast or in Ecuador, like Loja. The plague was recorded in Huancabamba and Ayabaca (in the highlands of Piura) between 1920 and 1930, and a rumour spread that there was pneumonic plague in Piura.[17] In Cajamarca, the plague began in the provinces closest to the coast, from whence migrant labour moved seasonally to the coastal rural estates. The mortality rate proved exceptional in this department: by 1916, 213 of the 351 cases recorded had died.[18]

The plague established its own circle of reinfection.[19] Coastal settlements spared by the first wave were exposed to infection when the plague spread from the ports to the countryside and the highlands. Due to the seasonal nature of the plague and the lack of resources, the people on the coast got used to the fact that the plague appeared with more or less intensity between November and March, that is, in summer, when the environmental conditions for the reproduction of rats increased.

How did Peru's people and authorities combat the plague, immersed as they were within a context which seemed to produce it? Several solutions were attempted in the first decades of the twentieth century. The first measure was taken when the plague extended from Callao to Lima, once the serious economic effects accruing from the disease were evident, and once fear had spread among the people.

Panic and the campaign in Lima

The plague arrived in Lima in late 1903. It caused panic and many fled. Rumours abounded which attributed all sudden deaths to the plague. Although it was unknown in the country, many could relate it to the apocalyptic stories of the plague in medieval Europe.[20] Even more worrying was the news that ships leaving Callao would not be received anywhere in the world, and that foreign ships would avoid Peru in order to evade quarantines. The result was a price rise in fares, mail, freightage and major commodities. It was a serious situation, for tariffs were one of the major sources of income for the government. According to one newspaper, prompt measures had to be taken because 'it is not just a matter of saving lives, but of saving our economic and fiscal interests'.[21]

An obstacle for the organization of a campaign against the plague was the lack of an efficient, country-wide sanitation system. The municipal governments, which were in charge of urban hygiene and the removal of refuse in streets, markets, slaughterhouses and homes since the late nineteenth century, and the welfare organizations which controlled hospitals and hospices, were swamped by critical conditions like those of 1903. The gap was partially filled by three new institutions: the Lima Municipal Institute of Hygiene, established in 1902, the Bureau of Public Health, which opened in 1903, and the Executive Board of the Campaign Against the Bubonic Plague in the Province of Lima, which was founded in early 1904.

The rise of these institutions was in part due to the sense of urgency an emergency creates, a factor that usually triggers legal and institutional changes in poor countries like Peru. The sanitary emergency found support in the climate of modernization that prevailed in Peru in the early twentieth century.

After its defeat in the War of the Pacific (1879–83), Peru underwent a period of economic growth based on the export of minerals, and reorganized a political élite which was represented by the Civil Party. This was a group of prominent lawyers, merchants and coastal landowners who began to rule on their own, after a period of military regimes, in 1903, the first year of the plague.[22] The political era that began a few years before, in 1895, with controlled elections is known as the 'Aristocratic Republic', and lasted up to 1919. The *civilista* élite deemed that the responsibility for the sanitary protection of ports and cities belonged to the State, and was a prerequisite for the progress of the export economy.

Although the Bureau of Public Health was created in response to the plague, its role went far beyond. The fear raised by a disease new to the country was used to establish the first nation-wide public institution in charge of public health. The organizations that preceded it in the nineteenth century were weak and did not command much respect. The Bureau was assigned to the newly established Ministry of Development, and had under its control all state physicians in charge of provinces, the lazarettos, the sanitary stations set up in ports, and the National Vaccination Institute, which was responsible for the production of the vaccine against smallpox. Although the Bureau did not have a distinguished role in the first years of struggle against the plague, it grew in importance and was the base on which a ministry in charge of health would be set up in 1935.

The Lima Municipal Institute of Hygiene was established shortly before the epidemic by the mayor Federico Elguera, a member of the *civilista* elite who was inspired by the institutes of hygiene established in all major European and Latin American cities since the late nineteenth century. Amongst other tasks, the institute had to manufacture serum and vaccines, supervise the medicines and foodstuffs sold, and analyse urine, blood, faeces and the milk of wet nurses.[23] Its first director was the Italian Ugo Biffi, who came to Peru specially hired by the municipality. Biffi repeatedly identified the plague bacillus in the bloodstream of the diseased, and organized sanitation campaigns in the provinces. His work consolidated in Peru the prestige of bacteriology and the germ theory of disease. Bacteriology, a field of study that developed in Europe from the 1880s onwards, and was taught in the University of San Marcos from 1895, eroded but did not end the miasmatic theories that ascribed the origin of infectious diseases to decomposing organic matter that entered the skin or the bloodstream. The National Academy of Medicine used bacteriological know-how when it formed a commission that confirmed the nature of the plague through the analysis of liquids taken from the lymph glands of the diseased, where the *Pastereulla pestis* bacillus was found.[24]

The institution that received the most publicity during the epidemic was the one established on a more ephemeral basis: the Executive Board of the Campaign Against the Bubonic Plague in the Province of Lima. Organized like the other Boards in the nineteenth century, it was financed by the State and was composed of representatives from the government, the municipality, a private charity institution in charge of hospitals known as the Beneficencia Pública and the Lima Chamber of Commerce.[25] Juan B. Agnoli, a prominent Italian physician who was Inspector of Hygiene in the Elguera administration, was named president and treasurer of the Board.

The appointment of Agnoli shows the need of conferring the power to carry out radical sanitation measures on a respected and experienced citizen. Educated in the Bologna Faculty of Medicine, Agnoli arrived in Lima around 1887 and became one of the most important physicians in the Italian Hospital. His studies of hookworm and tuberculosis were published in *La Crónica Médica*, Peru's foremost medical journal at the time. Thanks to his talent, dedication, European education and connections with the Lima elite (he married an upper-class lady), Agnoli managed to attain in just a few years what most professionals always seek: the admiration and respect of their colleagues, and to be sought by a large clientele. This prestige allowed him to take rigorous and drastic steps. Agnoli was convinced that the disease could be controlled in a brief span if he was given enough funds and executive powers.[26]

The Board headed by Agnoli got to employ slightly over a hundred labourers in charge of inspecting homes, hunting rodents, taking the sick to the lazaretto, and burying the dead. Agnoli was also in charge of masons who stopped up the entrance to rats' nests, applied tar to socles, destroyed the partition walls and flat ceilings the rodents could come in through, and eventually demolished the buildings. A sanitation police force was also his responsibility, and was in charge of breaking down the people's resistance.[27] It should be pointed out that the priorities of the campaign were to identify cases, isolate the sick, and bury corpses rapidly. Notwithstanding their effectiveness, the war on rodents and the incineration and reconstruction of homes were not regarded as important.

The procedure usually followed on detecting a case of the plague was to take the patient to the lazaretto, isolate the kin and fumigate the dwellings with sulphur. Fumigation was quite popular since the late nineteenth century, due to the belief that the disease was in the air or impregnated in objects. The home of the patient was destroyed in extreme cases. The removal to the lazaretto was carried out in zinc wagons specially built by the municipality, the stretchers on which the sick were carried were burnt and those who died were buried rapidly in distant corners of the cemetery.

Agnoli established strict rules during the campaign, such as a ban on the household rearing of poultry, dogs, guinea pigs, rabbits and cats – out of fear that these animals would spread the disease – and the temporary closing of schools, churches, circuses and all other places where people gathered. These bans were a survival of outdated medical ideas, because by then it was known that no animal other than the rat was a permanent source of the plague, and that the major method of contracting the disease is through the fleas in rats (unlike the pneumonic plague, which is rarer in Peru and is caused by contact between human beings).[28] Prizes in cash were likewise offered to get the co-operation of the people. The municipality bought each dead rat at 5 soles, and a similar amount was paid when someone reported a person sick with the plague.[29] These measures did not last long because few cases were reported, and because dishonest, low-income people set up kennels to rear rats and sell them to the authorities. The panic caused by the plague and the measures that led to police control gave rise to various responses.

Social responses

Criticisms of the sanitary intervention were partly due to disagreements concerning the perception of health and disease. The plague arrived in a milieu where bacteriology was not dominant, and where it was unusual for medicine to have an impact on the daily life of the people. The memoir presented by the Piura State physician in 1903, praising hygiene and questioning the new discoveries made with the microscope, shows that bacteriology was challenged among the physicians themselves: 'It has not yet been established whether microbes ... are the ones that cause disease, or whether they are produced by pathological alterations in the organism.'[30]

The lack of an agreement concerning the cause of the disease gave rise to a series of treatments, soaps and medicines produced by chemists and quacks, which were sold as a release from the plague. Amongst the most prominent were the *Jabón Fénico*, which alluded to the name of an acid; 'Tanglefoot', which destroyed flies as well as preventing the plague from spreading; *Fernet Branca*, an alcoholic beverage that was taken as an aperitif before dinner; and the *Legía Anti-Bubónica*, which besides being a disinfectant refreshed the skin, cleaned the floor and killed all kinds of insects.[31] The permanent advertisements for these remedies in the newspapers suggest that the people accepted them. The distribution of Haffkine's serum and Yersin's vaccine, which the Board promoted, stirred a debate. Members of the Board were charged with profiting because these items were relatively expensive, were imported from France, and were sold in a drugstore belonging to one of the inspectors from the municipality.[32]

The people at large did not believe that the plague was caused by microscopic organisms, or that it was necessarily mortal. It was thought that the plague was not deadly because buboes suppurated and dried up once a patient reached convalescence, and the death of a patient was frequently ascribed to the application of the anti-plague serum.[33] Domestic and traditional medicine had their own explanations. In Cajamarca there is still an oral tradition – perhaps dating to the beginning of the twentieth century – that regards the plague as an evil individual that is not to be insulted or hindered. According to this tale, a girl found the plague disguised as a woman dressed in black who took sheep away from her corral, but decided not to accuse her. The plague later returns the sheep and the girl does not fall sick. In Cajamarca, too, Indian groups used medicinal herbs against the plague, which were credited with having 'extinguished' the disease in places like Niepos.[34]

The serum and the vaccine promoted by the authorities were rejected not just due to cultural reasons. The anti-plague serum remained a controversial topic right until the 1920s because it proved useless after the fifth day of illness, and because the death rate in those treated with it was not significantly better *vis-à-vis* those who had not received it. Haffkine's vaccine produced a fever, swellings and other crippling reactions for a couple of days. It was because of these effects that the vaccine stopped being used in 1935. The serum and the vaccine were thus resisted by the people, and there were occasions when they had to be 'vaccinated by force'.[35] Another reason that explains the resistance shown to the measures was the roughness with which the sick were treated. The search for cases hidden by relatives and the compulsory isolation crossed the conventional frontier between the public and the private spheres. The sanitary intervention sponsored by the municipality and the State appropriated the care of the sick, something that had traditionally belonged to the family. This resentment surfaced in an article by the anarchist writer Manuel González Prada: 'Nothing more sacred than the bedroom, but not even this is respected. At the slightest indication of a plague, municipal agents assault sleeping quarters ... [and] examine the owner to ascertain if the bubonic strokes are rearing their heads in any of his glands'.[36]

Protests were also due to negligence and because it was believed that sanitation measures worsened the economic damage wrought by the plague. Specially important was the opposition owners made to the incineration of their property. Milne Mill, the focus of the epidemic, is a case in point. The news that a ditch was being dug around it for the cremation stirred the protest of the English stockholders of the mill and of the British consulate. The protests extended to Chile, from whence came a great part of the wheat and flour for the mills of Lima and Callao. To stop the measure, the interested parties questioned the very existence of the plague and held that the workers in the mill had died from suffocation. Opposition grew even though the Board agreed to pay for the premises. The merchants feared an interruption in the wheat trade and did not want to lose their mill, which had recently been thoroughly reconditioned.[37] The pressure exerted by the owners prevailed in the end, and prevented the measure from being applied with the convincing argument that it made no sense to burn the premises when the epidemic had already spread.

The most common reactions against medical intervention were individual and family ones, like denying the disease, hiding some cases, fleeing affected areas and the lazarettos, and an occasional minor revolt.[38] One of the most resisted measures was the disinfection and incineration of premises.

Incineration was a measure that sprung from the quest for immediate and dramatic measures in the most destitute provinces. Incineration was necessary for the State physician of Chota, in Cajamarca, because 'the huts', made of adobe bricks, mud and with earthen floors, would not admit any 'disinfection [other] than fire'.[39] An Incinerating Board was established in the port of Paita in 1905, which appraised and paid for the houses burned with funds from the office of the Prefect, using experts and keeping records. The local physician complained that this was only a temporary solution, for the owners would rebuild their homes in the same unhygienic conditions.[40] Incinerations played a symbolic role far beyond their usefulness, as they were spectacular and showed the authorities were 'doing something'.

This symbolic role extended to disinfections, a measure that was resisted because it ruined the furniture and other articles in the homes. A newspaper in Piura complained that the steps taken in the provinces were 'cosmetic', and added that 'the municipality believes it has accomplished its task by sending four men to clean up a rubbish heap somewhere, whereas there are another hundred more elsewhere'. It also defined disinfections as 'a spot of water with some drops of creosote left ... and nothing more'.[41] It should be borne in mind that disinfection was not much use since the buildings were in a state of dilapidation. According to the sanitarians themselves, it was no use having masons block up the lairs of rodents because these 'do not take long ... to open new entrances'.[42] *El Comercio*, the most important newspaper in Lima, pointed out the generalized presence of rats and criticized the compulsory measures taken because 'we would have to pray heaven to let loose a rain of disinfectant over the city'.[43]

Provincial officials had few resources to battle the worst ravages of the epidemic. For instance, in 1906 a State physician sent to San Gregorio, in Cajamarca, found many 'abandoned houses' due to the death of entire families.[44] In 1908, the physician in the province of Chota complained that the materials to fight the plague in Niepos came from Lima a month late, so he was forced to witness 'unmoved the death of those stricken'.[45] In this same department there were other manifestations of the dearth of resources. In 1923, the department's physician described thus the awful conditions in a remote locality in the province of Chota that had a population of 5000: 'a circle of death surrounds Huambos, and the materials we had for the campaign are running out'. This same report described the conditions in which he sometimes had to work:

> So far I have vaccinated 1,037 individuals and every day I visit the rural estates from 8 am to 9 pm, and each day I weigh the work that is left. The rains do not stop, it is no longer roads that I go through but mud puddles and soapy slopes, where life is endangered by the duty I have and will continue to set myself, until these places are cured.[46]

Supplies or physicians could not be sent to distant places, and so the work relied on vaccinators or improvised 'assistants' or 'inspectors' (medical students or people who had received basic training) who were paid a small salary and were equipped with serum, syringes, disinfectant and rat poison. Even some physicians did not know how to use all of these materials, as is pointed out in a letter the director of the Bureau of Public Health sent in 1909.[47]

The limitations of sanitation and the symbolic role of disinfections and incinerations were more marked in provinces where municipalities did not have enough resources for environmental sanitation, received the materials to fight the plague late and in insufficient amounts, and had the same tasks as the prefects. The latter headed the ill-defined Departmental Health Boards established in 1887, and which had an erratic existence until 1922. These Boards included in their budget an item called 'to fight epidemics', in recognition of future events.[48] In Lima it was considered that these Boards should financially support the municipalities, but local authorities thought an additional governmental subsidy for sanitation was needed. The officials in Lima eventually agreed to this even though the government only had scant funds in the budget for country-wide sanitation expenditures. It was only in the early twentieth century that the municipalities began to form a small bureaucracy, with aldermen specialized in collecting taxes, organizing expenditures, and having inspectors, including one for hygiene. Municipalities requested what they considered was essential for a campaign: financial resources and military support. A physician in Sullana, in the department of Piura, declared that no real sanitation campaign could be carried out 'without the help of a great many soldiers'.[49] Another typical case was that of Chiclayo, which had in 1908 a small budget for hygiene-related expenditures that was used up in the first months of each year.[50] The lack of resources made some municipalities tackle the war against the epidemics as a routine task, which had to yield some control without providing any long-term solution.

In other areas, the fears raised by the plague ensured that more attention was now paid to sanitation, and made some municipalities fulfill their role in environmental sanitation. To prevent the plague, in 1904 the mayor of Chiclayo urged the inspector of hygiene to burn rubbish, disinfect the streets, pressure farmers to clean the waterways, and post and distribute broadsides warning of the disease.[51] In 1908 a newspaper in Ferreñafe, in the department of Lambayeque, likewise pointed out that 'small puddles' which 'contaminated' the atmosphere formed when summer came, and that these should be eliminated to prevent the plague from spreading.[52]

Resistance to sanitation measures was dramatic when it came to identifying the sick. The zinc wagon in which these were moved in Lima cast a dark shadow and was popularly known as 'the death wagon'. The driver, a 'tough Indian' who lived in the lazaretto, often had to drive his cart through a crowd that threw stones at him. The fears worsened because some patients died before reaching the hospital. (According to Agnoli, these deaths were due to the serious condition of the patient, and to the ruggedness of the road.)[53]

In many localities, popular resistance also grew because the relatives and neighbours of the sick were held as 'suspect'. These were isolated in special houses, where they complained of 'great hardships and inconveniences'.[54] An editorial in *El Comercio* requested that the rigours of isolation be relaxed for the wealthy, and that 'those stricken with the disease' should remain in their homes 'when they have in them the means to be cared for'.[55] This same editorial overturned the preventive priorities of the government and demanded that removal to the lazaretto should be 'a measure for the protection of the sick, and not of the healthy'.

The flight and concealment of the sick was an option associated with the poor. San Gregorio, in Cajamarca, proved to be an extreme case where the officials and the people agreed to deny the existence of the plague to the government in Lima, and thus prevent their isolation.[56] A more typical one was that of the district of Catacaos (Piura), which was mostly inhabited by Indians and where many cases were 'concealed'.[57] The poor also confronted the government, as happened in the popular neighbourhood of Malambo, Lima, in March 1904. Neighbours crowded and vainly tried to prevent the removal of a sick child to the Lazaretto. According to a policeman, these incidents had to be avoided because 'the day will come when [the incidents] reach such magnitude that they shall become worse than the disease itself'.[58]

The efforts made to preserve social order led to the establishment of regulations for flight from infected areas. Sixty per cent of the 4500 inhabitants of the port of Mollendo migrated to the city of Arequipa with the support of the local authorities.[59] In Pacasmayo – where the first case of the plague appeared in 1903 – the physician sent by the government allowed migration as long as there was strict screening. More than 200 families from this port thus departed.[60]

Another area where the government and the people clashed was in the case of rapid burials, without any ritual and in conditions which caused apprehension, with the bodies wrapped in a blanket dipped in a strong disinfectant, buried 2 metres below the surface in zinc coffins and with 25 pounds of quicklime on top of them. This measure was resented by those who considered the cult of their dearly beloved as one of their major rituals. It was usual for the wakes to last for several days, waiting for the visit of relatives who lived in distant localities. When it was over, the deceased's clothes were washed and distributed among the participants, thus becoming a source of infection.[61] A typical case of resistance was the wake for Gregoria Lazo de Saavedra, who died in Catacaos on 21 February 1911. This lasted for three days despite the municipal order for a prompt burial, and the coffin was defiantly carried through the streets of the city accompanied by a music band and over 500 people.[62] The authorities were far more flexible in other provinces and allowed the wakes to take place at home, but restricted funeral corteges.[63]

Another image that fed popular fears were the lazarettos. The Lazareto de Guía was built on an arid plain on the northern entrance to Lima. Built of wood, it was surrounded with wire and steel fences, had several locks on the doors and was permeated by the smell of phrenic acid. With their dark shirt, raised collar, rubber boots and cap, the physicians in the hospital projected an image of command and asepsis. The Lazaretto had two pavilions for men and two for women, some of which were for paying patients. These had to take a salty purgative, follow a strict diet of milk and some medicinal herbs, and were weak – 'emaciated', according to an appropriate, contemporary expression – by the time they reached convalescence. For many, to recover from the plague was akin to a prelude to new ailments like tuberculosis, that preyed on exhausted organisms.[64] Those physicians who doubted the efficacy of these measures had to confront the Lazaretto nuns, who were intransigent as far as diet was concerned.

Popular fears of the Lazaretto rose due to the mortality among the patients isolated there, which officially reached the high number of 52 per cent in 1903–05.[65] Many believed it was higher and that secret burials were being made in non-consecrated grounds. A medical dissertation pointed out that for workers and peasants, entering the Lazareto de Guía was the prelude to death. Many times, 'the employees [had to] wage real battles with the incoming patients at the doorway'.[66] Rumours of clandestine burials were common in several provinces (by the mid-1920s there were seven lazarettos on the coast). A provincial newspaper described the popular perception of lazarettos: 'they are torn from their home and the company and care of their family, to be imprisoned in a hall ... [where the patients are] left to die on their own and ... be buried like dogs'.[67] An informant in Paita recalled tales of clandestine burials where bodies were cast into newly dug trenches, a story that hints at the fear inspired by the authorities:

> They went round all the streets of Paita and on hearing a moan ... marked the door with a cross and the gendarmes came in, removing whoever was sick with the plague ... this official [the head of the squad] was very evil because he threw a man sick with the plague into a ditch, and these ... while still alive sometimes begged not to be killed and asked to be healed, then this man threw a shovelful of earth over them and suffocated them.[68]

The resistance shown by the people and the weak medical resources used to fight the plague reinforced authoritarianism. The emergency committees established to control the plague were pressured to achieve immediate results. Physicians believed that only the strict enforcement of the health regulations would stop the disease. In the provinces, the people wavered between praising this control and criticizing it. This attitude was also combined with the demand for more government intervention, like in Ferreñafe, where a newspaper article demanded that 'they do not let us die like dogs ... and if the municipal revenues are due to the efforts of everyone, then nothing is fairest than to use them to look after the contributors'.[69] Although it is not easy to find sources which are openly critical of the authoritarian approach against the poor, a newspaper in Paita was eloquent enough:

> I detest the terror you inspire, the sanitary tyranny you exert in the name of your fantasies, your speculations, your hygienic mistakes. Centuries and centuries will evidently go by without you knowing the cause behind the transmission of diseases. You make theories others will destroy ... you will only ... [terrorize] the people, ruining trade, oppressing the proletariat [destroying] its homes and leaving the poor begging for alms ... For modern physicians do not need to heal, their sole occupation is being sanitary police agents! ... he who gets sick is a delinquent.[70]

The responses given to the epidemic did not just question authority. They also showed fault lines running down the entire social fabric, and revealed the fears felt by social and ethnic groups, and by individuals who lived in the same urban area. In normal times, these groups could carry out a more or less autonomous life, but some felt threatened by the sanitary crisis.

The plague and society

Since most of the sick came from poor neighbourhoods, the plague ended up being considered as a typical lower-class disease. According to the data for the Lazaretto of Lima, a high proportion of the patients did heavy manual work in the street and at home (journeymen, masons and day labourers, 81 cases; washerwomen and servants, 47; butchers and other food sellers, 47). These occupations come to 61 per cent of the 286 patients isolated in the Lazaretto, out of a total of 386.

Of all the cases, 252 were men and 134 women. Of the 386 patients treated in the Lazareto de Guía until January 1905, 186 were Indians and 65 were mestizos, that is, 65 per cent of the total. This does not indicate any kind of racial susceptibility, but rather the connection between low income and scant access to medical resources. If we make a breakdown of the mortality in the Lazareto by race, which was 47.9 per cent of all those interned, we find that while only 31 per cent of white patients died, 50 per cent of the total number of Indians did not survive. An even more terrifying figure is that of the Chinese, 92 per cent of all those who fell sick died.[71]

The very pejorative names by which the patients were called in Spanish – *pestosos* or *apestados*[72] – heightened the negative connotation and the stigma against filth and disease. Denying the plague was thus a way of distinguishing oneself from social groups and living conditions held as inferior. In other words, the denial was not just out of fear of isolation and fumigation; the disease was also associated with misery, poor living conditions and, even worse, with being Chinese or from the highlands – the scum of the earth for some. The authoritarian attitude sometimes shown by the sanitary authorities and the police gave rise to a connection between disease and crime. The plague was perceived as something that had to be hidden not just to avoid cures one did not believe in, but out of shame.

Physicians deplored the fact that in the affluent families of Lima, the 'rich would rather die of riches' hiding their plight, than admit they had fallen prey to the plague.[73] The doctors in the Lazaretto complained that although there were special wards for affluent people, these preferred being looked after in their home, and most of the paying sick were Italian and Japanese immigrants. The examination of passengers embarking in Callao is one sign that the authorities themselves believed there was a difference by social class. The Director of Public Health explained the characteristics of the examinations to the shipping companies:

> With first-class passengers, the inspection will be circumspect, trying to avoid as many inconveniences as possible ... particularly for the ladies; in general ... it shall be limited to an external examination, the condition of the tongue, pulse and temperature ... As many inconveniences as possible shall also be avoided with second class passengers too ... but vigilance shall be greater with them, since it is easier to find the sick among them.[74]

Public health was also apprehended as an instrument of social control and urban embellishment. A 1904 municipal decree banned beggars from passing through the city of Piura, most of whom came from Catacaos, an Indian town which had been strongly assailed by the plague. In an assumption that was no more than a prejudice, the beggars were believed to be 'germ-carriers' of the plague.[75] The significance of the decree was emphasized in 1907, for 'many beggars' bore the germs of 'disgusting diseases', and because 'this way, at least, this social plague is hidden if not extirpated'.[76] The adoption of other measures that segregated the popular sectors disclosed the racial prejudices present in Peru. One manifestation of this racism was blaming the Chinese for the epidemic. A significant Asian migration began to arrive in Peru from the mid-nineteenth century to work in the coastal rural estates, in guano extraction and on the railways, where they were treated almost like slaves. Around the turn of the century, the Asians lived in the most miserable conditions in the worst neighbourhoods. The Asians were the ethnic group which had most recently migrated *vis-à-vis* the other races, the one most easily distinguished by their appearance, culture and language, and the group with the least defence against the epidemic.

In many places it was believed that the plague had been caused by the Chinese. For example, in Callao the source of the epidemic was attributed to the Chinese cook Manuel Hubi, even though the first one to fall sick had been Pedro Figueroa. Hubi was actually the sixth case amongst the workers of the Milne Mill.[77] Likewise in Paita, one witness recalled that the plague began when two Chinese men were found dead inside a shop. According to this source, a crowd pillaged the shop and spread the plague throughout the city. Lastly, in Lima the police always suspected they would find plague cases in the homes and shops of the Chinese.[78] The miserable living conditions of the Chinese contributed to the association established between race and disease. Otaiza was one of the most famous *callejones* in downtown Lima. According to a 1900 article, inside it were:

> Chinese people in rags, packed one over the other, smelling of opium and filth; men lying all over, trying to sleep as best they can; sick and squalid bodies, half-wrapped in disgusting rags ... a bevy of filthy people who ceaselessly cough, thus filling the atmosphere with tuberculosis microbes which join the many others issuing forth from the people and the objects packed in this permanent focus of infection.[79]

The connection between the Chinese and the plague sparked a series of bills and legislative debates on Asian immigration. The alarm was sounded in October 1904 when a group of Chinese workers arrived at Callao, for it was believed they were bringing diseases with them. One senator even tried to ban the migration of Asians to Peru.[80] His project was long debated, and ended with a bill stating the 'danger' could be avoided with strict sanitary inspections. A far more stringent measure was taken in 1905, when a 'sanitary passport' was demanded of Asian immigrants because they were 'a confirmed danger to health'. These measures were part of a general debate on sanitation and migration. According to the most conservative position, the migration desired was European; the immigration of 'other races' caused serious economic, social, and hygienic problems. Part of the medical élite agreed with this position, as shown by an editorial in *La Crónica Médica* lamenting the hiring of Chinese workers, because this was the 'lowest [rung] ... of the human races'.[81]

The connection between disease and the 'Asian race' consolidated political beliefs that Peru was not doing enough to promote European migration, but was receiving the wrong kind of immigrants instead, and that the presence of epidemics was due to ignorance, as well as to the inborn characteristics of marginalized ethnic groups.[82] Although the prejudice against the Chinese decreased or was no longer so evident in later years, the custom of blaming disease on the idiosyncrasy of the lower classes would prove lasting.

Conclusion

The official response to the plague gave rise to a greater health intervention by the State, as the establishment of the Bureau of Public Health clearly indicates. Other indicators are the creation of lazarettos in all major cities, sanitary stations in ports, the widespread disinfections and several health regulations, including one for railways in 1904.[83] With these measures, local authorities and the people themselves were more careful with hygiene. This led to a reduction – at least transitory – in some diseases. A physician in the Municipality of Lima ascribed the general fall in mortality in 1903–04, particularly in tuberculosis, to the improvement in sanitation after the plague.[84]

However, these achievements were short-lived or insufficient. When in 1906 Agnoli made an appraisal of the epidemic in Lima, he admitted that the plague followed 'a marked trend to become endemic'. Something that caught his attention was that the number of rats caught was always about the same. He ascribed this to the economic constraints of the campaign, the ignorance of the people, and to urban living conditions where the reproduction of rodents was directly related to their destruction: 'As long as mountains of fermenting rubbish are just a few metres away from the most populated neighbourhoods; as long as people live huddled in humid, narrow and unclean *callejones*; as long as unseemly and hygienically unfit materials are used in buildings, it will be useless to talk of sanitation.'[85]

This extract reflects the predicament many doctors faced during an epidemic – either to allay the crisis with control measures, or to promote a preventive campaign to improve dwellings, rubbish collection, and environmental pollution. Agnoli himself wondered whether it had been worthwhile fighting the disease in a milieu where it was going to survive. His affirmative reply was based on humanitarian reasons, that is, in trying to prevent sickness and death. The work done by Agnoli during the epidemic is one example of the tragic circumstances many physicians in poor countries find themselves caught in.[86] Agnoli endangered his life, lost part of his clientele (who feared contagion) and saved valuable lives, but he could not prevent the spread of the disease. Although he received tributes and homages, Agnoli returned to Italy in 1910, but we do not know if he went through necessity or because he was disillusioned.

Like Agnoli, other physicians used the few resources available to face adversity with exemplary sincerity. One was Julián Arce, the director of the Bureau of Public Health, who asked the prefects to warn the people of the plague, and so 'make them know the danger in its true dimension; without exaggerations … or harmful and even more dangerous understatements'. Bearing in mind the social context, Arce distributed copies of a primer promoting conferences on the plague in schools, churches, army barracks and workers' meetings, where it was stated it was 'very important [that] Quechua be used [wherever] the Spanish language is not commonly spoken'.[87]

The plague was a problem for many years, especially on the north coast. Until the 1920s, the campaigns against the plague were sporadic, routine, symbolic and limited to times of crisis. This changed in the 1920s, when the Leguía administration adopted a series of measures for environmental sanitation. Of these, Law 4126, passed in May 1920, was especially important. It enabled the government to hire private companies to execute health projects in Lima and 32 other cities. The bill authorized the spending of $50 million on roads, sewers, pavement of streets, waste-disposal systems, safe water and to refurbish the ports. These were all built by the Foundation Company, which lent the government the funds at a 10 per cent interest rate.[88]

Furthermore, several decrees were passed in 1922 which, in a clear reference to the plague, established that buildings should have concrete foundations, prohibited walls made of wattle and daub on the ground floor, and empty spaces in floors, walls or between buildings, and conferred the power to authorize the construction of new urban areas to the Board of Public Health. Although never fully enforced, these and other regulations made life harder for rodents in urban environments.[89] The Technical Office of the Bureau of Public Health was established in 1925, when Lima was experiencing another wave of expansion, and it tightened control over buildings. At the national level, docks were refurbished with anti-rat measures, the use of concrete and asphalt was extended, and the water and sewage systems were improved.[90]

In 1930, a determined campaign to eradicate the plague from Peru was begun. The initiative came from the Pan American Sanitation Bureau (later the Pan American Health Organization), which sent the North Americans John D. Lang and C.R. Eskey to create the National Anti-Plague Service, train specialized personnel, and organize the manufacture and distribution of rat venom and traps. The campaign, financed by the Pan American Health Office, was extended to all localities which had had plague outbreaks in the five preceding years, and had as its major method the distribution of poison, although eventually some cents were paid for every rat caught. These measures, in conjunction with better environmental conditions brought about by the Leguía administration, drastically lowered the mean number of monthly cases. While there were more than 51 cases a month during 1920–30, the average fell to 16 cases a month for all of Peru in the first six months of the 1931 campaign.[91] The plague sporadically appeared between 1932 and 1936, and increased in the 1940s in some provinces, until DDT was applied.

The significance of the plague does not lie just in the 20 269 cases which appeared in 197 Peruvian localities in 1903–30. The number was probably higher because many had no medical assistance (Long estimated that there were 42 000 cases of plague between 1903 and 1930).[92] The true legacy of the plague was that it changed the attitude that the State, physicians, and part of the urban poor had towards public health. From the time of the plague onward, doctors increased their until then meagre participation in public matters. The epidemic was a great opportunity to convince public authorities and part of the population, of the importance methods and specialists in the area of hygiene had. What had until then been an act of charity from charitable societies or a routine task of the municipalities, now became a matter of state, requiring specialized institutions and detailed regulations.

Sanitary intervention was also understood by some as an activity controlling the inborn-leanings of the poorest people (like filth, ignorance or overcrowding), which could eventually become dangerous for the rest of society.[93] Some began to consider public health as a matter that had to be taken seriously, at least during epidemics, to protect their activities, reinforce their identity, and distinguish themselves from other groups. In the years that followed, the official response to epidemics consolidated the stigma associated with some infectious diseases, and reinforced the connection between physicians and power.

Notes

1. Juan B. Agnoli, 'La peste en Lima, Informe que eleva a la Presidencia de la Junta Directiva de la Campaña contra la Peste Bubónica en la Provincia de Lima', *Boletín del Ministerio de Fomento*, **2**, 1906, p. 3.
2. On the plague, see R. Pollitzer, *Plague*, World Health Organization, Geneva, 1954; Kenneth Kiple (ed.), *Cambridge World History of Human Disease*, Cambridge University Press, Cambridge, 1993, pp. 628–31.
3. Manuel Tamayo and Benjamín Mostajo, 'Cremación y utilización de la basura de Lima', *La Crónica Médica*, **409**, 1906, pp. 1–6.
4. Julio Ribeyro, *Saneamiento de Lima*, Imp. Gil, 1935, pp. 13–14; Luis Gómez, 'Sobre la peste bubónica en Sullana, Febrero 8, 1919', *Boletín de la Dirección de Salubridad Pública*, 1919, 128–33, La Opinión Nacionál, Lima, 1919.
5. Carlos Cisneros, 'Monografía de Lima', *Boletín de la Sociedad Geográfica de Lima*, **26**, 1910, p. 179.
6. *Prontuario de Legislación Sanitaria del Perú* (4 vols), Imp. Americana, Lima, 1937, 3, pp. 42–5.
7. Ramón Ribeyro, 'La peste en Mollendo', *El Comercio* (*EC*), 25 October 1903, pp. 2–3.
8. 'Informe del Médico Titular de Paita acerca de la peste bubónica durante agosto de 1905', in *Registro Oficial de fomento, Dirección de Salubridad Pública*, La Opinión National, Lima, 1905, pp. 171–2.
9. Juan A. Portella, 'La higiene en las casas de vecindad, necesidad de construir casas higiénicas para obreros', Bachelor thesis, Universidad Nacional Mayor de San Marcos, 1903, pp. 28–9.
10. 'Casas de vecindad', *EC*, 24 May 1903, p. 2.
11. Agnoli, 'La peste en Lima', p. 2.
12. Ibid.
13. Peru had more cases of plague than any other Latin American country right up to 1930. Arístides Moll and Shirley Baughman O'Leary, 'Plague in the Americas, Peru', *Boletín de la Oficina Sanitaria Panamericana*, **20**, 1941, p. 700.
14. In septicemic plague, an acute form of the bubonic plague, the bacillus invade the bloodstream and cause death before the buboes appear. Pneumonic plague begins like the bubonic plague and is complicated by pneumonia. It spreads when people inhale the sputum of a sick person. Eighty-six per cent of the 940 cases of the plague in 1904 were bubonic ones, and only 3 per cent pneumonic. Luis McNulty, 'Contribución al estudio de la peste en el Perú', Bachelor thesis, Universidad Nacional Mayer de San Marcos, 1912, p. 18.
15. Moll and Baughman O'Leary, 'Plague', p. 700.

16. The plague existed in Cajamarca since the turn of the century. *Director de Salubridad to Prefecto, 14 February 1913*, Serie Prefectura Cajamarca, Subserie Ministerio de Fomento, Leg. 221, Years 1913–20, Archivo Departamental de Cajamarca, Cajamarca (ADCa).
17. 'La Organización de los servicios sanitarios en el Perú', *Boletín de la Dirección de Salubridad Pública*, 1927, p. 23; Arquímedes Ramos Díaz, 'Epidemiología de la peste bubónica en la sierra del departamento de Lambayeque', *Boletín de la Oficina Sanitaria Panamericana*, **17**, 1938, pp. 776–81; Atilio Macchiavello, 'Estudios sobre la peste selvática en América del Sur, III', *Boletín de la Oficina Sanitaria Panamericana*, **44**, 1958, pp. 484–512.
18. *Director de Salubridad to Prefecto, 22 November 1916*, Serie Prefectura Cajamarca, Subserie Ministerio de Fomento, Leg. 221, Years 1913–20, ADCa.
19. *Prefecto to Director de Salubridad, 18 October 1917; 9 September 1920 and 12 July 1922*, Serie Prefectura Cajamarca, Subserie Libros Copiadores de la Prefectura a los Ministerios, Leg. 659, Years 1916–22. For Hualgayoc and Contumazá see *Director de Salubridad to Prefecto, 30 September 1921 and 10 October 1921*, Serie Prefectura de Cajamarca, Subserie Ministerio de Fomento, Leg. 222, Years 1921–29, ADCa.
20. The first person sick with the plague in Lima was Cirilo Rojas, a young Indian who worked near the slaughterhouse. Julio Boza, 'Contribución al estudio de la peste bubónica', Bachelor thesis, Universidad Nacional Mayor de San Marcos, 1916, p. 5.
21. 'Editorial', *EC*, 14 September 1903, p. 2.
22. Rory Miller, 'The Coastal Elite and Peruvian Politics, 1895–1919', *Journal of Latin American Studies*, **82**, 1982, pp. 97–120; Manuel Burga and Alberto Flores Galindo, *Apogeo y crisis de la República Aristocrática*, Rickchay Peru, Lima, 1980.
23. Jorge Basadre, *Historia de la República del Perú* (11 vols), Ed. Universitaria, Lima, 1969, 7, pp. 3413–59; Hermilio Valdizán, *Los Médicos italianos en el Perú*, Comité Pro-cociera Nell'America Latina, Lima, 1924, p. 174.
24. The plague microbe was known since 1894. Manuel Artola, Julián Arce and Daniel Lavorería, *La peste bubónica: Informe Presentado a la Academia Nacional de Medicina*, Imp. Torres Aguirre, Lima, 1903. For Peruvian bacteriology see Marcos Cueto, *Excelencia científica en la periferia, actividades científicas e investigación biomédica en el Perú, 1890–1950*, Tarea, Lima, 1989, pp. 120–26; For Ugo Biffi, see his *Saneamiento de Lima,* Imp. Gil, Lima, 1903.
25. Agnoli, 'La peste', p. 3.
26. Valdizán, *Médicos italianos*, pp. 133–6; 'Agnoli, Juan B.', in Hermilio Valdizán, *Diccionario de la medicina peruana* (3 vols), Talleres Larco Herrera, Lima, 1923, 1, p. 50.
27. Agnoli, 'La peste', pp. 54–5.
28. 'La situación sanitaria', *EC*, 10 May 1903, p. 2; John Long, 'Cooperative Campaign for the Eradication of Plague in Peru', *Public Health Report*, **31**, 11 September 1931, p. 2164.
29. 'La situación sanitaria', *EC*, 10 May 1903, p. 1.
30. Emilio Espinoza, 'Memoria del Médico Titular de Piura, 1903', *Registro Oficial del Departamento de Piura*, 20 March 1904, pp. 2–3, Archivo Departamental de Piura, Piura (ADP).
31. Advertisements in *EC*, 27–28 May 1903, p. 1.
32. *Prontuario*, 3, pp. 591–2.

33. *Prefecto to Director de Salubridad, 22 March 1906*, Serie Prefectura Cajamarca, Subserie Libros Copiadores de la Prefectura a los Ministerios, Leg. 655, Years 1904–11, ADCa. Víctor Pérez, 'Algunas consideraciones relativas a la etiología, patogenia, tratamiento y profilaxia de la peste en Lima', Bachelor thesis, Universidad Nacional Mayor de San Marcos, 1923, p. 70.
34. Statement made by Segundo Manosalva Huañambal, La Camaca, in *Los Hombres de Kishuar, la medicina en la tradición cajamarquina*, Aspaderuc-PEC, Cajamarca, 1991, pp. 76–7. *Director de Salubridad to Prefecto, 20 February 1909*, Serie Prefectura Cajamarca, Subserie Ministerio de Fomento, Leg. 220, Years 1909–12, ADCa.
35. *Director de Salubridad to Prefecto, 22 November 1916*, Serie Prefectura Cajamarca, Subserie Ministerio de Fomento, Leg. 221, Years 1913–20, ADCa. Thomas Butler, *Plague and Other Yersinia Infections*, Plenum Medical Books Co., New York, 1983, p. 198. Gómez, 'Sobre la peste', p. 131.
36. González Prada, 'Nuestros licenciados Vidriera', in Manuel González Prada, *Horas de lucha*, Ed. Universo, Lima, 1972, p. 173. The article was originally published in 1903.
37. 'El molino mandado quemar' 'La peste reconocida oficialmente' and 'La bubónica en Iquique', *EC*, **9**, 28 May 1903, pp. 1, 2, and 4 respectively.
38. According to the police, while officials looked for the sick person in one house, relatives took the patient to another. *Subprefecto de Policía to Prefecto, 29 March 1904*, Fondo Ministerio del Interior, Prefectura Lima, Subprefectura Lima, Leg. 16, Year 1904, Archivo General de la Nación, Lima (AGN).
39. *Julián Arce to Nicolás Hernández, 1 April 1909*, Serie Prefectura Cajamarca, Subserie Ministerio de Fomento, Leg. 220, Years 1900–12, ADCa.
40. 'Informe del Médico Titular', pp. 171–2. 'Libro de Actas, Junta Incineradora, Tasadora y Pagadora, principiado el 5 de agosto de 1905', Archivo Municipal de Paita, Piura (AMPa).
41. 'La peste y los apestados', *El Sol*, Piura (*ES*[P]), 4 February 1915, p. 1.
42. Agnoli, 'La peste', p. 38.
43. 'En la Municipalidad', *EC*, 6 April 1904, p. 2.
44. The physician's report in *Prefecto to Director de Salubridad, 22 March 1906*, Serie Prefectura Cajamarca. Subserie Libros Copiadores de la Prefectura a los Ministerios, Leg. 655, Years 1904–11, ADCa.
45. The State physician was *Nicolás Hernández writing to Julián Arce, 8 December 1908*, and *Director de Salubridad to Prefecto, 9 February 1909*, Serie Prefectura Cajamarca, Subserie Ministerio de Fomento, Leg. 220, Years 1900–12, ADCa.
46. *Augusto Maradiegue to Prefecto, 8 April 1923*; and *'Resumen de los datos para el censo general de la república proporcionados por los gobernadores y subprefectos del departamento de Cajamarca', 12 December 1918*, Serie Prefectura Cajamarca, Subserie Libros Copiadores de la Prefectura a los Ministerios, Leg. 659, Years 1916–22, ADCa.
47. *Director de Salubridad to Prefecto, 27 February 1923*, Serie Prefectura Cajamarca, Subserie Ministerio de Fomento, Leg. 222, Years 1921–29, Dirección de Salubridad, *'Requisitos para desempeñar los cargos de inspector sanitario o vacunador, junio 6, 1924'*, Serie Prefectura Cajamarca, Subserie Ministerio de Fomento, Leg. 222, Years 1921–29, ADCa.
48. *Director de Salubridad to Prefecto, 10 March 1916*, Serie Prefectura Cajamarca, Subserie Ministerio de Fomento, Leg. 221. Years 1913–20, ADCa.
49. Gómez, 'Sobre la peste', p. 132.
50. *Alcalde to Prefecto, 5 December 1908*, Concejo Provincial de Chiclayo, Archivo

Alcaldía, Libro Copiador de Comunicaciones, Years 1906–12, Archivo Departamental de Lambayeque, Chiclayo (ADLa).

51. *Alcalde to Inspector de Higiene, 6 April 1904*, Concejo Provincial de Chiclayo, Alcaldía, Libro Copiador de Comunicaciones, Years 1904–06, ADLa.
52. 'Focos de infección', *El Grito del Pueblo*, Ferreñafe (*EGP*), 1 January 1908, ADLa.
53. 'Carros para apestados', 'En el Lazareto de Guía', *EC*, 30 May 1903, p. 3, and 30 October 1904, p. 4; and Agnoli, 'La peste', p. 27.
54. E. Congrains, 'Una opinión atendible', *EC*, 11 April 1904, p. 2.
55. 'Editorial', *EC*, 14 April 1904, p. 1.
56. *Prefecto to Director de Salubridad, 22 March 1906*, Serie Prefectura Cajamarca, Subserie Libros Copiadores de la Prefectura a los Ministerios, Leg. 655, Years 1904–11, ADCa.
57. 'Concejo distrital de Catacaos', *Biblioteca Municipal de Piura*, Piura (*BMP*), **58**, 15 April 1909, p. 1, ADP.
58. *Subprefecto e Intendente de policía to Prefecto, 30 March 1904*, Fondo Ministerio del Interior, Prefectura Lima, Subprefectura Lima, Leg. 16, Year 1904, AGN.
59. Ramón Ribeyro, 'La peste en Mollendo', *EC*, 25 October 1903, pp. 2–3.
60. 'La peste en Pacasmayo', *EC*, 8 November 1903, p. 2.
61. Nazario Chávez, *Cajamarca* (2 vols), Talleres Leoncio Prado, Lima, 1957, 2, p. 211.
62. 'Alcalde de Piura a Presidente de la Junta Distrital de Sanidad, febrero 23, 1911', *BMP*, **5**, 15 March 1911, p. 11; 'La peste negra', *EGP*, 15 January 1910, p. 3, ADLa.
63. 'Inspección de higiene', *El Progreso* (Chiclayo), 15 September 1911, p. 1, and *Alcalde to Prefecto, 18 March 1911*, Concejo Provincial de Chiclayo, Archivo Alcaldía, Libro Copiador de Comunicaciones, Years 1906–12, ADLa.
64. Aníbal Odicio, 'Contribución a la seroterapia de la peste', Bachelor thesis, Universidad Nacional Mayor de San Marcos, 1911; Luis Amorín, 'Mi experiencia personal en la campaña contra la peste', Bachelor thesis, Universidad Nacional Mayor de San Marcos, 1930.
65. Segundo Ortega, 'La peste en el Perú, desde su aparición hasta 1924', Bachelor thesis, Universidad Nacional Mayor de San Marcos, 1925, p. 2.
66. Amorín, 'Mi experiencia', p. 36.
67. 'La peste y los apestados', *ES*(P), 4 February 1915, p. 1; 'Carrozas sospechosas', *La Prensa*, 7 April 1904, p. 8. *Subprefecto to Prefecto, 22 March 1904*, Fondo Ministerio del Interior, Prefectura Lima, Subprefectura Lima, Year 1904, Leg. 16, AGN.
68. Jaime Abad Coloma, interview with the author, Paita, 21 September 1989.
69. 'La peste negra', *EGP*, 15 January 1910, p. 3, ADLa.
70. 'Espanto sanitario', *La Igualdad*, 13 March 1906, p. 2, AMPa.
71. Juan B. Agnoli, *Memoria elevada a la Alcaldía por el Inspector de Higiene del Concejo Provincial de Lima, La Peste Bubónica en los años de 1903 y 1904*, Imp. Gil, Lima, 1905, pp. 8–9.
72. Offensive terms that emphasize the smell of plague-stricken people.
73. Amorín, 'Mi experiencia', p. 52.
74. *Director de Salubridad to Agente de la Compañía de Vapores, 13 April 1904*, Serie Prefectura Cajamarca, Subserie Ministerio de Fomento, Leg. 220, Years 1900–12, ADCa.
75. *'Prohibición del ingreso de mendigos de Catacaos a esta ciudad, 1911'*,

Expediente Municipal, Year 1911, p. 17, Archivo Municipal de Piura, Piura (AMPi).

76. J.A. Atkins, 'Erogación para mendigos', *BMP*, **1**, 1 June 1907, p. 2; 'Junta Provincial de Sanidad', *BMP*, **6**, 15 March 1912, p. 128; ADP.
77. Artola, Arce and Lavorería, *La peste*, p. 6.
78. Jaime Abad Coloma, interview, 21 September 1989; *Subprefecto e Intendente de Policía to Prefecto, 24 February 1904*, Fondo Ministerio del Interior, Prefectura Lima, Subprefectura Lima, Leg. 16, Year 1904, AGN.
79. 'En los garitos', *EC*, 8 July 1900, in *El siglo XX en el Perú a través de 'El Comercio', 1901–1910*, El Comercio, Lima, 1991, p. 274.
80. Basadre, *Historia*, 7, p. 3456.
81. 'Los coolis'; 'Inmigración de asiáticos, Lima, julio 21, 1905', in *Prontuario*, 1, p. 73.
82. For this approach see Enrique León García, *Las razas en Lima*, Sanmartí y Cía., Lima, 1909.
83. *Director de Salubridad to Capitán del Puerto, 30 March 1904*, Serie Prefectura Cajamarca, Subserie Ministerio de Fomento, Leg. 220, Years 1900–12, ADCa.
84. Portella, *Datos demográficos*, p. 3.
85. Agnoli, 'La peste', p. 73.
86. Agnoli received a thousand pounds and a gold medal, Cámara de Diputados, *Diario de debates, Congreso Ordinario de 1904*, El Comercio, Lima, 1904, p. 557.
87. *Director de Salubridad to Prefecto, 19 May 1904*, Serie Prefectura Cajamarca, Subserie Ministerio de Fomento, Leg. 220, Years 1900–12, ADCa.
88. Ministerio de Fomento, *Anales de las obras públicas del Perú*, Ministerio de Fomento, Lima, 1920, p. 300.
89. *Augusto B. Leguía, 29 September and 16 October 1922*. The documents were for all of Peru. *Sebastián Lorente to Prefecto, 2 December 1922*, Serie Prefectura Cajamarca, Subserie Ministerio de Fomento, Leg. 222, Years 1921–29, ADCa.
90. 'El problema de las basuras de Lima', *La Crónica Médica*, **80**, 1925, pp. 19–20; 'La Organización de los servicios', p. 16.
91. C.R. Eskey, 'Epidemiological Study of Plague in Peru', *Public Health Reports*, **47**, 18 November 1932, pp. 2191–207.
92. Ibid.
93. Rómulo Eyzaguirre, *La mortalidad de los lactantes de Lima, sus causas y sus remedios*, Imp. San Pedro, Lima, 1908.

CHAPTER TWO

Sanitation from Above: The Rockefeller Foundation and Yellow Fever

Yellow fever was considered one of the major plagues of the New World from the seventeenth to the early twentieth century. Tropical and subtropical cities in America, from New Orleans to Buenos Aires, were exposed to epidemics that diminished the population, paralysed trade and gave rise to a feeling of uneasiness and panic.[1] By the late nineteenth century, the fever seemed to vanish in Lima and the Peruvian coast, until an outbreak took place in 1919 that finally ended in 1922 with the intervention of the Leguía administration and the Rockefeller Foundation (RF). The campaign was directed by North American experts who had boundless confidence in technological resources, paid scant attention to the communitarian side of health, and were even less interested in educating the people. This chapter discusses the authoritarian nature of the efforts made to eradicate a disease that was held as a threat for the rest of the world, and reviews the adverse responses that combined the traditional resistance to sanitation measures (as had previously happened with the plague) with a more modern regional and nationalist opposition to foreign influence.[2]

Exterminating the fever

For many experts, the eradication of yellow fever was possible by the early twentieth century. This optimism was based on previous work carried out in 1900 by a US Army commission in Havana, which demonstrated that the fever was transmitted from a sick person to a healthy one by the *Aedes aegypti* mosquito. This species is rarely found far away from habitations, and mostly breeds in artificial water containers (unlike other mosquitoes such as those of malaria, which prefers lakes and ponds).[3] Shortly afterwards, William Gorgas ended the fever by ridding Havana of the *Aedes*; this convinced many others that the method would get the same results elsewhere. Gorgas himself applied this method against malarial and yellow fever mosquitoes in Panama, thus enabling the construction of the canal during 1904–14.

This optimism gave rise to the so-called Key-Centre Theory, on which several campaigns were based (including the one carried out in Peru). This theory held that the disease only attacked human beings, produced immunity in those who survived the first infection and was transmitted solely by the *Aedes aegypti*. According to this theory, the disease was likewise endemic in major ports and coastal cities (labelled key centres) which always had an important number of non-immune individuals (due to the permanent flow of migrants and visitors, and to natural growth). According to this approach, small urban centres did not pose a threat for bigger populations, and were always infected from outside. The practical implication was that the fever would automatically vanish if strong campaigns against the mosquito were carried out in the urban key centres, which were not many in the Americas.

The traditional methods used to fight mosquitoes included fumigation, covering water containers with wire mesh, isolating the sick, the quarantine of ports, the establishment of land sanitary controls isolating infected populations and the rebuilding of premises. These methods were expensive, complex and unreliable, so only the most powerful countries could apply them.[4] However, in 1910 the new theory received a new impulse when the campaigns focused on destroying the *Aedes* larvae in domestic water containers (the mosquitoes laid their eggs in these vessels). This approach lowered the costs and simplified the task as it reduced sanitation work to one single technique. It was believed that yellow fever would automatically vanish if the percentage of larvae dropped to about 2 per cent.

The International Health Board (later on the Division) of the Rockefeller Foundation was established in this optimistic milieu in 1913. The primary goal of this organization was to extend to the whole world the experience of the Rockefeller Health Commission, which had worked against hookworm in the southern USA. The eradication of yellow fever in American cities where it was endemic was added to this goal after 1916, partly due to the influence of Gorgas. Three factors were behind this decision: the fear that the endemic ports of South America would re-infect the southern USA with yellow fever; the risk that the Panama Canal (opened in 1914) would take the fever from the Caribbean to tropical Asia, which was free of the disease; and the pursuit of an American scientific triumph. The identification of the organism behind the fever, which would have helped develop serums and vaccines, seemed such an important objective that many US scientists went after it. These included members of the Rockefeller Institute of Experimental Medicine, a biomedical research centre sponsored by the RF.

The Foundation launched its first campaign against yellow fever in Latin America in July 1918, when it succeeded in controlling an epidemic outbreak in Guayaquil, a port that was held to be a focus of infection in South America. The campaign included a scientific commission from the Rockefeller Institute that tried to determine the etiology of the fever. A spectacular result achieved by Hideyo Noguchi, a member of the commission, was the identification of a micro-organism that caused yellow fever. Noguchi called it *Leptospira icteroides*, and on his return to the USA manufactured a serum and a vaccine for the disease.[5] Although neither was ever used as the major means of prevention and treatment, both were distributed and used by thousands of people in Latin America.[6]

The Key-Centre Theory and Noguchi's 'discoveries' gave rise to a feeling that the scientific and epidemiological aspects needed to control the plague had already been defined. For many experts, those of the RF included, all that was needed to achieve eradication was the rigorous application of some techniques. However, new discoveries made since the mid-1920s indicated that the Key-Centre Theory and Noguchi's discoveries were both wrong. These discoveries included: the transmission of yellow fever through several species of mosquitoes, the infection of wild monkeys living in the jungle, the presence of a jungle (sylvatic) variety of yellow fever (where the vectors belong to the genera *Aedes* and *Haemagogus*) and, above all, the fact that small communities do mantain an endemicity and can reinfect major population centres. Noguchi's studies on the fever were therefore wrong, and his serum and vaccine were both useless. In 1927, a RF laboratory in Africa determined that the fever was caused not by *Leptospira i.* but by a virus, and it was only in 1937 that an effective vaccine was finally available.[7]

In spite of these mistakes, the Key-Centre Theory was useful for the control of yellow fever in urban areas far removed from the forest, like the cities and ports of Peru. The campaign that the Foundation carried out on the north coast was directed against the mosquito that carried the disease. The Peruvian Foundation's participation was preceded by the work of a North American physician hired by the Peruvian government: Dr Henry Hanson.

A North American in Peru

A graduate of Johns Hopkins University, Hanson had been a professor of pathology in several North American universities, Director of the Bacteriological Laboratory of the Sanitary Office of the State of Florida, and a member of the US Public Health Service in the Panama Canal. When he was 39 years old, Hanson arrived in Lima in May 1919 with a rudimentary command of Spanish to study health conditions, with particular reference to malaria. Soon after his arrival he witnessed two events that suggested the country that he was in had trouble with authority: the workers' strike against the increase in the prices of major commodities, and the coup of Augusto B. Leguía.[8]

Reports of a 'mysterious' disease in Piura reached Lima before he finished his study. These were not taken seriously until the death rate rose rapidly. The Leguía administration then decided to send Hanson to identify and fight the epidemic. Hanson observed the typical symptoms of yellow fever, such as chills followed by a strong and violent fever, jaundice, cramps, dilated pupils, a red tongue, a fetid breath, nose haemorrhage, and yellow-coloured skin. He likewise observed that a dark-coloured liquid (coagulated blood) was vomited in the most serious cases. The disease had a definitive outcome. It was all over in about ten days, with the patient either dead, or recovering and henceforth immune to the disease. The symptoms led Hanson to establish that it was yellow fever, possibly introduced by a merchant who had come from Guayaquil. This first case spread the disease in a population that could not recall having had it since 1895.[9] The fever occurred in Paita, Sullana and Piura between June and November 1919. Ten more localities in the department were infected in the first half of 1920, and a total of 455 cases were recorded.[10]

The administration wanted to control the outbreak because Piura had an important role in the Peruvian economy. The rise of Piura's large rural estates for the export of cotton to the international market during the First World War was possible due to the expansion of the land under cultivation, either through the incorporation of uncultivated lands or through the encroachment on community plots, to the presence of available labour in a region known as Lower Piura, to technical improvements in the cultivation and watering systems, and to good maritime communications through the port of Paita.[11]

Paita, a magnificent bay with calm waters all year long, some 62 kilometres from the city of Piura, was a mandatory port of call for all ships sailing between Lima and Panama or Mexico, where major export houses and foreign consulates had opened. The economic importance of Piura was all the more remarkable because Lobitos and Talara, valuable oilfields worked by the American companies Lobitos Oilfield Ltd and the International Petroleum Company (the latter connected to the oil interests of the Rockefeller family), were located in the department. Catacaos, an Indian town with an important output of straw hats, skin and leather is 11 kilometres away from Piura.

Living conditions had not improved in Piura for most of the people, even though cotton had suddenly risen in price during the First World War. International demand encouraged the rural estates or *haciendas* to seize lands and direct their output to the international market, neglecting local demands. The poor living standards were revealed by the open-air sewage system, the proliferation of waste tips, the unhealthy conditions present in markets, the lack of toilets and a marked lack of water for domestic usage. These factors connived to expose Piura and the north coast to the blows of malaria, the plague, smallpox, dysentery and typhoid fever.

The campaign which Hanson led in Piura was in part based on traditional methods like fumigation, which is explainable because he had little experience with yellow fever. Hanson commanded a health squad to move the sick to a lazaretto, close the port of Paita, inspect the water supply to check if there were *Aedes a.* larvae in it, and reinforce the sanitary blockade formed by soldiers in the southern part of the Department to prevent flight by land. One measure that proved difficult to execute was the ban on meetings after 6 p.m., including those held in churches, cinemas, schools and circuses. Hanson banned them in the mistaken belief that meetings stimulated the dispersal of the disease. Fumigation, a costly procedure that only eradicated adult mosquitoes, proved frustrating because most buildings were made with hollow walls of wattle and daub, and the empty spaces here and in the roofs did not let the vapour concentrate.[12]

Neither was it easy to get the people to clean their water tanks daily, a step that would have eliminated the *Aedes aegypti* larvae. Water is one of the most valuable possessions on the dry north coast, and was carefully stored in clay vessels and other containers like earthen jars, short-necked jugs, filter stones, barrels and wells which held the water used to drink, wash, cook and for other assorted uses. Some containers were protected with metal mesh or had lids, but most did not and became the preferred breeding grounds for *Aedes*. According to a US observer, not 'one drop of water' was wasted in the area.[13] Since the water supply was scarce, Hanson designed a slow and unwieldy system to clean it: the liquid was filtered through a thin cloth, which let one identify the larvae.

The steps taken by Hanson faced stiff local opposition from physicians who questioned his diagnosis and methods, from merchants who resented the strict quarantine which forced ships to cancel their customary stop in the docks of Paita, from artisans who spurned the manned sanitary blockades established to control the transportation by land of passengers and merchandise, and from people who rejected fumigation because of the damage it inflicted on their property, hid their sick, and refused to renew their water containers more often.[14]

There was little Hanson could do with limited funds and scant personnel, who had no experience with yellow fever either. He himself contracted the fever before he finished his work and underwent the classic treatment, which included cold baths every four hours, purgatives and oranges and pieces of ice taken orally to offset vomiting. He survived. Hanson decided to return to the USA after recovering and had become immune to the fever – something he would always be proud of – but he was somewhat frustrated at not having completed his task. The Peruvian government asked him to carry out a more thorough health campaign on the north coast shortly before his departure. Hanson demanded a high salary and left, convinced that his request would be denied.[15] However, on arriving at Panama he got a cable that his demand had been accepted.

It was no mere chance that Hanson was hired anew by the Leguía administration (1919–30). Leguía believed that the development of Peru hinged upon the arrival of foreign capital and know-how. According to a US official, Leguía had admitted that he wanted to have a North American in charge of each branch of the government.[16] Leguía often showed his desire for US technical, commercial and financial help. Besides Hanson, Leguía also hired other North Americans to direct educational, agricultural and health activities, arguing that local resources were inadequate and had to be modernized. As was seen in

Chapter 1, in 1920 he also signed a contract for sanitation works in several cities, with the Foundation Company, an American engineering firm. These works reinforced the centralized form of government that characterized the Leguía administration. All were carried out under government supervision, with almost no participation from local authorities.

On his return to late-1920s Peru, Hanson found that yellow fever and other diseases had sparked epidemics in Piura and other coastal regions like Lambayeque. In Catacaos (Piura), severe epidemics of bubonic plague and fever were compounded by cases of smallpox, dysentery, typhoid and measles. However, Hanson decided he should focus on the plague and on yellow fever, as these were the most virulent diseases. At that time Paita, a town with a population of 3500 by 1920, also had a severe outbreak of the plague that eclipsed the importance of yellow fever. There were five deaths a day here for several weeks.[17] The bubonic plague was endemic in Paita and on the coast, as was shown in Chapter 1. In fact, the plague gathered strength again in the department of Piura between 1918 and 1923, with 960 recorded cases of which 339 were from Paita.[18] Besides the conditions described above in this town there was an additional factor that favoured the reproduction of rats: the fishermen used to keep dry fish beneath their beds. This made the rats build their lairs near the beds, and their fleas moved on to warmer bodies once the rodents died.

Hanson decided to apply a radical solution to eradicate the plague and the fever for good: the complete incineration and reconstruction of Paita. In defence of his proposal, he argued that only six houses could be 'refurbished' for 'human occupancy' according to US living standards.[19] His goal was not just to make the new houses rat-proof, but something he believed was more important: the transformation of Paita into an ideally healthy town that could be a model for the rest of Peru. The United States' involvement in the control of epidemic outbreaks in twentieth-century Latin America has usually been related to a desire to raise productivity and to eliminate the impact quarantines have on areas of export agriculture.[20] Hanson's plan indicates that yet another motivation behind this concern was the diffusion of a health model inspired by the living standards of urban North America, and reveals the messianic attitude brought by some foreigners who were trying to promote a radical transformation in Latin American public health.

William Gorgas was visiting Lima and had his doubts on the convenience of razing Paita to the ground, which he deemed was not essential. However, Gorgas and Leguía accepted Hanson's plan as a way of imparting a 'lesson' to the rest of the country.[21] The plan involved burning and rebuilding all the houses in Paita, reimbursing the owners for their lost property and relocating the families in barracks which would be sold to their occupants in instalments. The Foundation Company began tearing down the poorest quarters of Paita, but met with such resistance that only a few blocks – about 10 per cent of the town – could be burned.[22] It was because of this opposition, and partly because a ship from the US Navy entered Callao in late 1920, that Hanson interrupted his work on the north coast to organize a brief campaign against prostitution in Callao, and so 'prevent' the contagion of the North American visitors.[23]

The RF sent a new commission to Piura while Hanson was working in Peru, to confirm the findings Noguchi had made on yellow fever. This mission included Noguchi himself, Gorgas, and Colonel William D. Wrightson. In early 1921, the Foundation sent a cablegram to the Peruvian authorities offering resources to wage an intensive campaign against yellow fever.[24] Leguía immediately accepted, and in May 1921 Hanson was appointed Director of the campaign, and Wrightson Director of the Board of Public Health.[25] The first contribution made by the RF was US$5000, on condition that the Peruvian government would reimburse 50 per cent of the total cost of the campaign. When the campaign was over, Hanson had spent US$115 000 from the Foundation, but the administration had fulfilled the deal only in part.[26]

Leguía and the Rockefeller Foundation

The enthusiasm Leguía had for the Foundation's support can be explained not just by his desire to attract North American technicians, but also by his concern for the protection of a financially important area, as well as to consolidate his political influence. The fever had extended to Lambayeque, Leguía's homeland, and was threatening the department of La Libertad. The first was the most important rice-producer in Peru, the second, the major producer of sugar cane. Rice, a staple part of Peruvian diet, was grown in small and big estates, sheltered by protectionist legislation. The huge sugar estates of La Libertad whose output went to the world market, had expanded thanks to favourable prices during the First World War, when the European beet producers were forced off the market.

In both the departments of Lambayeque and La Libertad, the fever especially affected the workers who came to work at the coastal rural estates from the highlands. The traditional problem which coastal agriculture had of labour shortage, had been solved through the *enganche* system. This began in the late nineteenth century and persisted until the 1930s. It consisted in advance payments in merchandise or cash made to highland Indians from Cajamarca, La Libertad and Ancash, in order that they would work on the coastal *haciendas*. This compulsive way of acquiring labour was resisted due to the overexploitation it entailed, but also because of the 'physical [ravages] the changes in climate, food and work rhythm inflicted on them'.[27] It is worth pointing out that physicians were aware of the differential impact of yellow fever, as is disclosed by a letter the director of the Health Bureau sent to the prefect of Cajamarca, indicating that the disease could be contracted in the ravines close to the coast, while the 'high-altitude areas located in the midst of the highlands are free … from infection because [the *Aedes*] cannot easily develop there'.[28]

The health campaign in the north was also due to the pressure exerted by the major landowners or *hacendados*. The large sugar-producing rural estates had given rise to powerful landowners who controlled the Civilista Party, the major political association in the 'Aristocratic Republic'.[29] The effects of a political dispute between the *civilistas* and Leguía were still being ironed out during the yellow fever epidemic. The president had come to office thanks to a *coup d'état* in July 1919, after the inconclusive polls where he ran against the *civilista* candidate. Congress then confirmed and legalized his coup. The new president persecuted and deported his political rivals, and showed that he was firmly committed to retain power at all costs. Under his administration, the *civilista* leaders did not hold any position in the administration, but they retained their economic privileges and influence in northern Peru.

Leguía tried to extend the authority of the State in the provinces, questioning the traditional roles of local authorities such as hygiene. The campaign led by Hanson played an important part in the growth of the authority of the Leguía administration, eroded the power of provincial authorities and contributed to the development of a public health system. A decision that helped these goals was the centralization of public health and the growth of the civil service. In June 1922, Wrightson established the Departmental Health Bureaus run from Lima, as a replacement for the old Departmental Health Boards which were managed by the municipalities.[30] Shortly after the epidemic, the man responsible for health in the Leguía administration criticized the 'retrograde' and 'charitable' notion of medicine and welfare that he associated with '*civilismo* and the oligarchy', and applauded the efforts made by the government to construct public facilities which would yield a preventive and more vigorous public health.[31]

While legitimizing and extending its power, the Leguía administration developed an unprecedented relation between US health officials and the Peruvian State. Leguía relied on the economic, technical and scientific resources of the USA in order to implement health policies that would reaffirm his authority. Physicians in Lima and provincial institutions had a subsidiary and complementary role in the campaign. The authoritarian traits of the Leguía administration helped the kind of campaign Hanson wanted to develop. Hanson concentrated exceptional powers to prevent public opinion from hindering the sanitation policies, as had happened in his first term in Peru. A governmental decree placed him in charge of all sanitation activities from Callao to Peru's northern frontier. With this power, Hanson could command any steamer and place provincial physicians and authorities under his command. Eventually, he even had a cavalry regiment with 40 men and a cruiser docked in Paita. Hanson himself described his position thus: 'I have arranged an almost absolute autonomy (or dictatorship) in all matters pertaining to the campaign.'[32]

Hanson focused on the north coast because the clusters of towns located along the seasonal rivers, the small number of urban centres, the sparse population dispersed around the countryside and the valleys separated by desert areas, presented an ecology that helped the rapid dispersal of the fever. Areas with a certain population density provided an abundant food supply for *Aedes* and threatened to extend the fever to Lima and Callao, which had endured severe outbreaks of yellow fever in the nineteenth century. One of Hanson's major goals was to prevent the disease from spreading to the central coast area.

The work Hanson carried out with the support of the Rockefeller Foundation was characterized by an incomplete adherence to the Key-Centre Theory. The campaign focused on those localities with the highest population, whether they were infected by the fever or not, instead of on eliminating the epidemic in small localities even when these had a high death rate. Hanson justified this procedure which entailed abandoning small towns, with the lack of staff and his faithfulness to the Key-Centre Theory, which held that the fever would eliminate itself. He predicted that susceptible individuals would die or survive in the small localities, thus becoming immune, while the set number of births, visitors and migrants in the bigger urban centres constantly added to the population a significant number of susceptible individuals. So it was that a prophylactic campaign was carried out only in centres with a certain population density, or that were on a route that helped the disease disperse to non-infected areas. Many towns, hamlets and *haciendas* were therefore abandoned to the fever.

Hanson began to use the serums and vaccines developed by Noguchi with the help of the Foundation.[33] As was previously explained, it was shown by the late 1920s that the vaccine was useless and that those vaccinated with it could indeed contract the fever. However, more favourable results were obtained thanks to the experience acquired in the Rockefeller campaign in Guayaquil in 1918. Particularly important was an artful method that used river fish as larvaecides. After experimenting with six different species, Hanson noticed that small fish survived in domestic water containers eating *Aedes a.* larvae, were inoffensive to humans, and were abundant in the northern rivers. The most active larvaevores were the *mojarra*, the *chalcoque*, and especially the *life*.[34] This system surpassed all traditional methods of mosquito control like drainage, spreading oil on breeding grounds and the fumigation of adult mosquitoes.

The solution employed was simple – to capture and breed these fishes for their distribution in the water containers. Hanson distributed them from his headquarters in Chiclayo, the capital city of the department of Lambayeque, through a system that employed one hundred health workers. Towns were divided into districts under inspectors, labourers and sometimes children who visited houses and carried buckets of fish. The workers made weekly inspections examining water containers, roofs, holy water fonts in churches and other containers where liquids could be stored. The containers were emptied and cleaned when larvae were found, and the larvaevores placed in a new store of water. Hanson kept a detailed record of the expenditures made, the houses and buildings inspected, and the containers of water that had been treated.

At first some did not allow fish to be placed in their favourite jars, out of fear that the fish's excreta would taint the water. But the system was accepted shortly thereafter and became the most important measure taken during the whole campaign. What's more, it seemed to have a lasting effect as it was used for many years.[35] Seven hundred thousand home inspections were made in 1921, and a bigger number of fish was distributed.[36] Bearing in mind the limitations of fumigation and isolation, which used up energy and funds, and the defects of the water-supply systems, this simple, cheap and effective method was what practically eradicated yellow fever in northern Peru.

However, in mid-1921 the fever broke through an ineffective land quarantine and infected the department of La Libertad. By then the epidemic extended from southern Piura to the northern fringes of the department of Ancash.[37] The index of *Aedes a.* was high in this area, which included some hundred population centres: 60 to 100 per cent.[38] In the east, the advance of the epidemic was halted by the Andes, on whose elevations *Aedes a.* could not survive. The campaign in La Libertad controlled the fever in a short time thanks to the experience acquired, the assistance received from the Rockefeller Foundation and to the fact that the fever in this area was mild. By 1921 the worst of the epidemic was over, and Hanson announced that the index of *Aedes a.* had fallen to less than 3 per cent. By early 1922, Hanson was well in control in all towns north of the department of Lima, and no new case of yellow fever was reported.[39] At that moment Wrightson resigned his position as director of the Board of Public Health, and Hanson was named in his place until July of that year, when he returned to the USA. The RF left Peru at the same time.

Hanson estimated that a total of 15 000 cases of yellow fever had produced 1000 deaths during 1919–21. According to Hanson, most of the cases were concentrated in the department of Lambayeque, with a total of 10 000 cases. At the height of the epidemic, parts of Lambayeque like Olmos, Motupe and Ferreñafe each registered between 8 and 20 deaths a day. The figures given by Hanson are based not on the number of cases recorded, but on the assumption that these were a tenth part of the actual total.[40] Complete records were never kept because Hanson considered the campaign should concentrate on eliminating the larvae once the infection appeared in a town. It was likewise impossible to keep accurate records due to the cases hidden, because many managers in the rural estates refused to provide data, and because there was no way to ascertain the extent of the fever in many small hamlets which were known to have it. The figures given by Hanson are not surprising because the mortality of yellow fever is usually low, between 5 and 10 per cent in all cases.[41]

The Pacific coast of South America has remained free of yellow fever since 1922. The 1919–22 epidemic played a marginal role in the mortality of the north coast's urban population. It did, however, have an important role in bolstering the fear people from the highlands had of coastal diseases, laid bare the deficiencies in the sanitary infrastructure, and consolidated state intervention in provincial public health. The authoritarian campaign headed by Hanson produced antagonisms, resistance and open opposition that reflected individual fear of the disease, the prominent role of local authorities and the social tension caused by the changes that had taken place in the region.

Control and reactions

Hanson never managed to have most of the public co-operate actively with him. His diagnosis of yellow fever was met with some incredulity and, in some areas, like Trujillo, the health workers were forced to exhibit samples of black vomit kept inside a transparent glass.[42] Those who questioned his methods included the merchants, who were trying to avoid the restrictions placed on trade. The powerful Trujillo Chamber of Commerce firmly but mistakenly believed that Hanson was responsible for the decision taken by Panamanian authorities, to establish several days' quarantine for all steamers coming from Peruvian ports, and other merchants complained that many ships refused to get close to regions with the fever.[43]

For reasons of their own, many officials downplayed the epidemic and joined the opposition presented by the merchants. Several prefects and mayors considered that the arrival of a foreigner invested with power by the government in Lima was a violation of their authority, and resisted the loss of their political prerogatives. In June 1921 the prefect of Trujillo sent a telegram to the authorities in Lima saying he was 'construing the opinion of the department' that it was being 'damaged by the hasty declaration of yellow fever'.[44] Hanson had allowed the steamers to stop in infected ports but not to take passengers, and he defended himself saying that 'many people talk too much of a subject they know nothing about', and that the economic damage would be greater if drastic measures were not taken.[45]

A clear indicator of the resistance shown to some of the sanitation measures was the failure of the attempt to isolate the infected areas by land. The sanitary blockades established by Hanson were evaded or became sources of contagion, as happened with the one between Lambayeque and La Libertad, where the soldiers came down with the fever and fled south. Those who disobeyed the prohibition included not just people fleeing from the fever, but also pilgrims travelling to religious festivals and merchants or artisans out to sell their goods. Complaining of the scant value of land blockades, Hanson stated that 'If an influential individual comes along and offers the officer in charge of the squad five *soles* or a pound, it usually is "pasa señor" '.[46]

The most articulate opposition to Hanson came from the small but influential community of local physicians. Many of these doctors were concentrated in the cities, and their clientele came from the middle class and the upper echelons of society.[47] The few paid positions in public administration were part time and had low salaries. Local physicians did their best to discredit the diagnosis of yellow fever. They usually pointed out the absence of the classic black vomit, and diagnosed the fever as a serious case of malaria or blackwater fever, a condition that did not require the strict restrictions established by Hanson. These critiques confirm the lack of experience local physicians had with yellow fever, because vomiting only appears in severe cases, but also reflect the survival of other medical conceptions.[48] For some, the fever was an opportunity to establish heterodox connections between miasmatic conceptions and the germ theory of disease: this was caused by fetid airs given off by rotting animals and human waste. According to Dr Ugaz from Chiclayo, the fever was endemic in some parts of Lambayeque because these areas had a 'certain amount of heat' which facilitated the reproduction of mosquitoes, and because 'the wind did not disperse the mosquitoes' in some filthy and poorly ventilated neighbourhoods. Ugaz also took advantage of the epidemic to preach about the risk posed by alcoholism and the decomposition of poorly stored food which could worsen the epidemic, and advised that the best thing to do in the face of the crisis was to 'keep up the spirit'.[49]

Dr M. Eli Uceda, who published a series of newspaper articles against Hanson in *La Industria* (a newspaper in Trujillo) was a typical provincial doctor specialized in several ailments (ear, nose and throat, urinary tract, lady's ailments; general and surgical medicine). Uceda believed the proclamation of an epidemic in Trujillo to be exaggerated and hasty. He demanded a detailed clinical discussion on the origin, evolution and spread of the fever, and accused Hanson of wasting an immense budget. Critiques like that of Uceda reflected the way diseases were perceived by local physicians trained in a clinical perspective, who were used to consider a multiplicity of causes and accompanying infections, and who studied each individual case instead of the epidemiology of a whole population.

Paradoxically enough, the 'backward' local physicians used 'modern' bacteriology to support their arguments and undermine Hanson's diagnostic and preventive methods. Uceda pointed out that the causal agent identified by Noguchi, *Leptospira icteroides*, could not be found in the bloodstream of the sick, and so the epidemic could not be yellow fever.[50] This statement suggests that the correlation which is sometimes established between the successes of bacteriology and preventive medicine was not as direct as it seems, and that the first was perhaps also used to confirm paradigms that were apparently outdated. Moreover, the results attained by bacteriology could likewise be used as an argument that local doctors were using: the higher efficiency of local physicians over foreign ones when treating domestic ailments.

The campaign against fever also touched off some massive protests. One of them took place in February 1921 in Ferreñafe, a town serving small- and middle-sized rice farms a few kilometres from Chiclayo. One hundred and four cases of yellow fever, out of a population of 10 000, were officially reported in this town.[51] One of Hanson's assistants was sent to the area and prohibited pubic gatherings. The local doctor and the owner of a cinema protested, and a defiant parish priest celebrated a Mass that ended in a procession. A crowd of some 200 individuals then invaded the sanitary office and assaulted the employees of the campaign,[52] who barely had time to escape. The situation was still tense until the prefect sent a train full of troops. However, these were of little use for the fever broke out among the soldiers. Hanson then decided to leave Ferreñafe and place his forces 'where they would be more useful'.[53]

The strong nationalism prevalent among the workers and the middle class of northern Peru is another reason for the social protests against the sanitation campaign. This nationalism developed partly because the major sugar-producing landowners in one of the most influential valleys of the region, Chicama, in the department of La Libertad, were immigrants or foreigners.[54] Nationalism increased because profits and wages fell once the favourable prices brought about by the First World War were over.[55] A general strike swept the valley in 1921, in solidarity with the workers of one *hacienda*. The measure hindered Hanson's activities in the area. The strikers did not let the sanitary measures recommended by a 'yankee physician' be enforced in Casa Grande, the major Peruvian sugar *hacienda* in the 1920s, which employed 25 000 workers and was the property of a German corporation.[56]

According to Klaren, the history of confrontation between *hacienda* workers and immigrant owners contributed to the rise of the Popular Revolutionary American Alliance (APRA). By then a transition from the *enganche* system to a rural proletariat was beginning in the sugar estates. Many of the trade unions formed in the cane fields were integrated into APRA, which launched an active campaign against imperialism and social inequality. Some of its leaders, including Víctor Raúl Haya de la Torre, came from the middle-class families of Trujillo which had been ruined by the social dislocation brought about by modernization.[57] Considering the debate caused by Hanson's campaign in the newspapers of Trujillo, it can be argued that nationalist concerns in this area increased due to a perception of foreign intervention in hygiene. The campaign supported by the RF influenced the way workers drew the line between what was foreign and what was national.[58]

Hanson had his own idea of the relationship between the national and international interests involved in the campaign. With that same idealism that surely inspired his plans for the reconstruction of Paita, Hanson argued that over and above the local indifference and petty interests of the trade unions, there was one supreme goal which Peru should embrace or submit to – the eradication of yellow fever from the world. In an attempt to overcome the resistance of the strikers in Casa Grande (whom he considered 'Bolsheviks'), Hanson accused them of 'hindering a universal project ... that cannot be considered as a matter of concern only to Peru'.[59] The goal set by the Rockefeller Foundation entailed eliminating the epidemic from Peru and so break the international chain of transmission. This argument must have heightened the impression that the head of the campaign had a list of priorities prepared abroad, and must have sounded strange in an area where most people were used to living with high rates of tuberculosis, smallpox and other infectious diseases, and where the usual method of sanitarian intervention in an epidemic was merely symbolic.

Hanson actually made little effort to understand the nature of local opposition. From his point of view, there always were people who opposed sanitarian measures in all countries, and there was no sense in debating 'around matters that have been established and confirmed about 25 years ago'.[60] An editorial in a Trujillo newspaper complained of the silence and arrogance of the North Americans: 'Dr. Hanson insists on doing us good in his own way. He gives us no explanation because these take too long.'[61] An even stronger article criticized the unproductive 'autocratic system' of sanitation.[62]

Hanson envisaged the struggle against fever as a demonstration of modern techniques coming from developed countries, and of the experience of tropical medicine in an age focused on eliminating the vectors of infectious diseases.[63] Due to the reductionist view then prevalent in tropical medicine, the campaigns carried out in various parts of the Third World were begun under the assumption that in a 'backward' and non-scientific culture, the disease should be handled with little regard for the perceptions and opinions of the patients. The adverse reactions of the people were treated as an atavism that had to be set aside. Paradoxically enough, Hanson's haughtiness and his claim to authority supported by western science, which would hardly have been effective without the support of Leguía and the Rockefeller Foundation, were based on scientific errors like the Key-Centre Theory and Noguchi's *Leptospira*. In the 1930s it was concluded that the fever could not be eradicated, and that a partial control and protection through immunization were more realistic goals. As a result, the RF abandoned its eradication campaigns and Hanson's work was seen as a successful episode, albeit without any major epidemiological significance because it was part of a mistaken scientific design.

Conclusion

When Hanson wrote his memoirs of the three, intense years he lived in Peru, he called them *The Pied Piper of Peru*. The title was a metaphor between a medieval tale where a piper frees a town from rats, and one of the most dramatic events in the campaign – the attempt to burn Paita to free it of the plague. The book presents a doctor who used modern techniques to fight an epidemic alone and unsuccessfully. Furthermore, it shows a physician who loved an ideal and his work more than the sick; a doctor who passionately strived to attain an ambitious sanitarian goal designed by the Rockefeller Foundation, often going beyond what the people could accept and what the Foundation and Gorgas himself suggested: caution. It is possible that Leguía and the Foundation had material and humanitarian interests in wanting to prevent the ravages of the fever. However, for Hanson the campaign was an opportunity to test his character, a chance to become one of the medical heroes who eliminated a disease and a chance to set an example for international sanitation.

His vision, at times overly romantic, and his unlimited confidence in techniques did not win him any sympathy, and instead caused disapproval and resistance. His frustration, and that of other US doctors who took part in the campaign, did nothing to redeem the negative reputation of native society. This perception transferred the blame for the disease onto the people without questioning the labour systems, living conditions, or the lack of a sanitarian infrastructure. In his memoirs, Hanson wrote: 'Supertitious, ignorant and seemingly satisfied, the rank and file of the natives of Lambayeque, as everywhere in Peru, were resentful of any effort to direct or change their mode of life'.[64] Inspired by the sight of a cemetery with the victims of yellow fever, a North American assistant of Hanson's wrote a poem which reflected the conflict between the doctors and the people:

> Shame, Shame to those who daily fought
> The knowledge that science so dearly brought,
> Nor lifted a hand to save a life,
> But added fuel to the fires of strife,
> The battle is won and the Gringo fain
> Would return to the land, from whence he came.[65]

The limitations inherent to this kind of sanitarian campaign began to be evident in the 1930s. The romantic age of foreign doctors who wiped out epidemics with radical methods alone and rebuilt public health in tropical countries, was now over. However, something remained of Hanson's campaign. From the 1920s onward, US influence and government intervention in public health began to be more evident. This intervention was characterized by proposing technically contained solutions that paid scant attention to the environmental, cultural and communitarian factors behind the disease. On the other hand, the unlimited reliance on the power of some techniques served to control the worst epidemic outbreaks, but it was not the only way of responding to the lack of health resources, as is shown in the following chapter.

Notes

1. Henry Carter, *Yellow Fever: An Epidemiological and Historical Study of its Place of Origin*, Williams and Wilkins, Baltimore, 1931. Donald B. Cooper and Kenneth Kiple, 'Yellow Fever', in K. Kiple (ed.), *The Cambridge World History of Human Disease*, Cambridge University Press, Cambridge, 1993.
2. The rise of nationalism on the north coast has been associated with the origins of the Alianza Popular Revolucionaria Americana. Peter Klaren, *Modernization, Dislocation and Aprismo: Origins of the Peruvian Aprista Party, 1870–1932*, University of Texas Press, Austin, 1973.
3. Nancy Stepan, 'The Interplay between Socio-economic Factors and Medical Science: Yellow Fever Research in Cuba and the United States', *Social Studies of Science*, **8**, 1978, pp. 397–424; William Coleman, *Yellow Fever in the North: The Methods of Early Epidemiology*, University of Wisconsin Press, Madison, 1987, pp. 13–20; W.G. Downs, 'History of Epidemiological Aspects of Yellow Fever', *Yale Journal of Biology and Medicine*, **55**, 1982, pp. 179–85.
4. 'La fiebre amarilla, medios de evitarla', *Boletín de la Dirección de Salubridad Pública*, 1919, pp. 37–41.
5. Paul Clark, 'Hideyo Noguchi, 1876–1928', *Bulletin of the History of Medicine*, **33**, 1959, pp. 1–20; Lois Parks and Gustave Nuermberger, 'The Sanitation of Guayaquil', *Hispanic American Historical Review*, **23**, 1943, pp. 197–221.
6. *Heiser to Flexner, 12 July 1920*, Rockefeller Foundation Archive (RFA), R.G. 5, Series 1.1, Box 47, Folder 713, Rockefeller Archive Center, New York (RAC).
7. Coleman, *Yellow Fever*, p. 11. Some believe that Noguchi confused yellow fever with Weils' disease. See E. Bendiner, 'Noguchi: Many Triumphs and a Brillant Failure', *Hospital Practice*, **19**, 1984, pp. 222–7; The RF produced the first effective, wide-scale vaccine by 1940, Greer Williams, *Virus Hunters, The Lives and Triumphs of Great Modern Medical Pioneers*, Alfred A. Knopf, London, 1960, pp. 124–5.
8. Henry Hanson, *A Study of Sanitary Conditions in Peru with Special Reference to the Incidence of Malaria*, Panama Canal Press, Mount Hope, 1921; Henry Hanson, '*Informe general sobre el estudio de las condiciones sanitarias del Perú durante tres años, 1922*', RFA, R.G. 5, Series 2, Box 36, Stacks 331, RAC.
9. Manuel Quirós, 'Demostración de la vía que ha seguido la fiebre amarilla al invadir el norte del Perú', *La Crónica Médica*, **38**, 1921, p. 400. José Toribio Polo, *Apuntes sobre las epidemias en el Perú*, Federico Barrionuevo, Lima, 1913.
10. Carlos Enrique Paz Soldán, *La sanidad pública en el Perú*, Imp. Torres Aguirre, Lima, 1920, pp. 19–25.
11. Susana Aldana and Alejandro Díez, *Balsillas, piajenos y algodón, procesos históricos en Piura y Tumbes*, CIPCA, Lima, 1994, p. 101.
12. José Alván, 'La fiebre amarilla en Tamarindo y Catacaos', Bachelor thesis, Universidad Nacional Mayor de San Marcos, 1920; Carlos E. Zapata, 'La fiebre amarillaen Piura', Bachelor thesis, Universidad Nacional Mayor de San Marcos, 1920.
13. William C. Gorgas, *Diary, 18 September 1919*, RFA, R.G. 12.1, RAC.
14. 'A título de saneamiento', *La Industria*, Piura (*LI*[P]), 4 May 1920, p. 2.
15. *Gil Cárdenas a Prefecto de Lambayeque, 21 May 1921*, Serie Prefectura Lambayeque, Subserie Ministerio de Fomento-Dirección de Salubridad, Año 1921, ADLa.
16. *J.A. Sterling to Secretary of State, 29 November 1921*, Records of State Relating

to Internal Affairs of Peru, 1910–29, Political Affairs, Microfilm Roll 4, National Archives, Washington, DC (NA).

17. Henry Hanson, *The Pied Piper of Peru: Dr. Henry Hanson's Fight Against 'Yellow Jack' and Bubonic Plague in South America, 1919–1922*, Convention Press, Jacksonville, 1961, p. 57.
18. Atilio Macchiavello, 'Estudios sobre peste selvática en América del Sur, II', *Boletín de la Oficina Sanitaria Panamericana*, **43**, 1957, p. 226; Atilio Macchiavello, 'Estudios sobre peste selvática en América del Sur, III', *Boletín de la Oficina Sanitaria Panamericana*, **44**, 1958, p. 484.
19. Henry Hanson, 'La campaña sanitaria en Piura', *EC*, 16 May 1920, p. 8; Henry Hanson, 'The Sanitation of Paita', *West Coast Leader*, **9**, 436, 1920, p. 2.
20. Richard Brown, 'Public Health and Imperialism: Early Rockefeller Programs at Home and Abroad', *American Journal of Public Health*, **66**, 9, 1976, pp. 897–903; Saúl Franco Agudelo, 'The Rockefeller Foundation's Antimalarial Program in Latin America: Donating or Dominating?', *International Journal of Health Services*, **13**, 1, 1938, pp. 51–7.
21. Gorgas, *Diary, 18 March 1920.*
22. The barracks were demolished in the early 1970s because they had become the most unhealthy area in Paita. Abad Coloma, interview, 21 September 1989.
23. *Ministro de Fomento a Ministro de Gobierno y Policía, 22 December 1920*; and *Gil Cárdenas a Prefecto del Callao, 22 December 1920*, Fondo Ministerio del Interior, Prefectura Lima, Paquete 213, Year 1920, AGN.
24. *Leguia to Gorgas, 14 January 1920*, RFA, R.G. 5, Series 1.2, Box 97, Folder 1336, RAC.
25. J.A. Estrella Ruiz, 'La sanidad peruana en cincuenta años: Apuntes para su historia', *Salud y Bienestar Social*, **6**, 1953, p. 92.
26. *William H. Wrightson a Director del Tesoro, 15 February 1922*, Fondo Ministerio de Fomento, Dirección de Salubridad Pública, Leg. 810–136. Año 1922. AGN. '*Statement of Money Deposited with the Equitable Trust Company of New York by the International Health Board and Checks Drawn on this Account in Peru by Henry Hanson, up to March 31st, 1922*', RFA, R.G. 5, Series 1.2, Box 139, Folder 1836, RAC.
27. Wifredo Kapsoli, 'Movimientos sociales en Cayaltí, 1915–1919', *Allpanchis*, **11**, 1978, p. 106.
28. *Director de Salubridad a Prefecto de Cajamarca, 3 November 1921*, Serie Prefectura Cajamarca. Subserie Ministerio de Fomento, Lima, Doc. 737, Leg. 222, Years 1921–29, ADCa.
29. Manuel Burga and Alberto Flores Galindo, *Apogeo y crisis de la República Aristocrática*, Rickchay Perú, Lima, 1980.
30. 'La Organización de los servicios sanitarios en el Perú', *Boletín de la Dirección de Salubridad Pública*, 1927, p. 15.
31. Sebastián Lorente, 'La Obra médico social del gobierno del señor Leguía', *Boletín de la Dirección de Salubridad Pública*, 1927, p. 137.
32. *Hanson to W. Rose, 17 March and 6 June 1921*, RFA, R.G. 5, Series 1.2, Box 117, Folder 1573, RAC.
33. Two reports list the names and age of 526 individuals from La Libertad, inoculated with the Noguchi vaccine. '*Relación de las personas inoculadas con la vacuna Noguchi en Trujillo*'; '*Relación de personas inoculadas con la vacuna Noguchi en Paiján, 23 September 1921*', RFA. R.G. 1.1, Series 331, Box 3, Folder 18, RAC.
34. *Aequidens rivalatus*, *Lebiasina bimaculata*, and *Pudigium punctulatum*,

respectively. International Health Board, *The Use of Fish for Mosquito Control*, Rockefeller Foundation, New York, 1924, p. 52.

35. In September 1989 I found that the system was still in use in Motupe and Monsefú, two towns near Chiclayo, to control malaria and other diseases. In May 1995, the students in a course on the history of health in Lambayeque confirmed that this procedure is still used in the area.
36. Hanson, '*Preliminary Report on the Recent Yellow Fever Epidemic in Peru, 1922*', RFA, R.G. 5, Series 2, Box 36, [No folder], RAC.
37. *Hanson to Robert Kirk, 15 April 1921*, RFA, R.G. 5, Series 1.2, Box 117, Folder 1573, RAC.
38. Hanson, *Pied Piper*, p. 124.
39. *Hanson to Reed, 4 August 1921*, RFA, R.G. 5, Series 1.2, Box 117, Folder 1574, RAC.
40. *Hanson to Rose, 5 April 1921*, RFA, R.G. 5, Series 1.2, Box 117, Folder 1573, RAC.
41. George Strode (ed.), *Yellow Fever*, McGraw-Hill, New York, 1951, p. 397.
42. Amador Rosales, 'Algunas consideraciones profilácticas observadas en la epidemia de fiebre amarilla en Paiján', Bachelor thesis, Universidad Nacional Mayor de San Marcos, 1924, p. 7.
43. *Agustín Ganoza to Alfredo Pinillos, 29 January 1921*, Correspondencia Recibida, Years 1921–22, Archivo de la Cámara de Comercio de Trujillo, Trujillo (ACCT). *Hanson to W. Pareja, 18 May 1921*, RFA, R.G. 5, Series 1.2, Box 117, Folder 1573, RAC.
44. *Telegrama from Prefecto to Presidente de la República, 24 June 1921*, RFA, R.G. 5, Series 1.2, Box 117, Folder 1573, RAC.
45. *Letter of Hanson to comandante H. Herrera, prefecto, 25 June 1921,* RFA, R.G. 5, Series 1.2, Box 117, Folder 1573, RAC.
46. *Hanson to Rose, 18 June 1921,* RFA, R.G. 5, Series 1.2, Box 117, Folder 1573, RAC. 'Cómo cumple su función el cordón sanitario', *La Reforma* (*LR*), 8 March 1921.
47. 'La fiebre amarilla en Ferreñafe: reportaje al Dr. Pagador', *LR*, 4 February 1921.
48. Luis G. Tapia a Junta Departamental de Sanidad, 22 April 1921, in Rosales, 'Algunas consideraciones', p. 12.
49. Dr Ugaz, 'Fiebre amarilla, vómito negro', *El Tiempo*, Chiclayo (*ET*), 21 January 1921, p. 2, ADLa.
50. *LI*(T), 5 May 1920, p. 3. The following articles by Uceda appeared in *LI*(T): 'Algunas consideraciones sobre el presunto caso de fiebre amarilla', 11 May 1921, 1, p. 4; 'El problema de la fiebre amarilla, duplica al médico sanitario', 15 June 1921, p. 1.
51. *J.H. White to Rose, 27 September 1921*, RFA, R.G. 5, Series 1.1, Box 56, Folder 812, RAC.
52. *L. Chuman to Prefecto de Chiclayo, 24 January 1921*, Concejo Provincial de Ferreñafe, Libro de Correspondencia, Years 1920–21, ADLa.
53. *Hanson to Rose, 25 May 1921*, RFA, R.G. 5, Series 1.2, Box 117, Folder 1573, RAC. 'El estado sanitario de Ferreñafe, motín del pueblo contra los médicos', *LI*(T), 4 February 1921, p. 2.
54. Carlos Bachman, *Departamento de Lambayeque, Monografía Histórico Geográfica*, Imp. Torres Aguirre, Lima, 1929, p. 242.
55. Michael González, *Plantation Agriculture and Social Control in Northern Peru, 1875–1933*, University of Texas Press, Austin, 1985, p. 176.
56. Hanson, *Pied Piper*, p. 131.

57. Uceda used nationalist arguments to oppose 'foreign' sanitation. 'La salubridad en Trujillo, las restricciones sanitarias son absurdas e innecesarias', *LR*, 20 July 1921, p. 2.
58. Roy MacLeod and Milton Lewis (eds), *Disease, Medicine and Empire Perspectives on Western Medicine and the Experience of European Expansion*, Routledge, London, 1988.
59. *Hanson to Rose, 24 September 1921*, RFA, R.G. 5, Series 1.2, Box 117, Folder 1574, RAC.
60. Hanson, 'El problema de la fiebre amarilla', *LI*(T), 16 June 1921, p. 2.
61. 'La dictadura amarílica', *LR*, 18 June 1921, p. 2.
62. 'El manifiesto de ayer', *LR*, 15 June 1921, p. 2.
63. According to Uceda the campaign was one-sided because it concentrated on the mosquito and had little concern for the sick. Uceda, 'A propósito de la fiebre amarilla, apostillas a la exposición del director de la campaña antiamalírica', *LI*(T), 18 June 1921, p. 2.
64. Hanson, *Pied Piper*, p. 107.
65. Ibid., pp. 111–12.

CHAPTER THREE

Public Health and the Community: Epidemic Typhus and Smallpox in the Andes

The events discussed in the previous chapters were marked by collective suffering, a lack of resources and authoritarianism. However, this was not the whole story. There were also cases of community involvement, the promotion of hygiene according to pre-existent cultural configurations, and a kind of silent heroism. This happened in Puno in the 1930s, where other ways of understanding and controlling disease appeared which reflected the influence that social ideas had on medicine, the steadfastness of Indian culture and the creativity of some individuals.

The department of Puno was the stage for an experiment that combined native medical beliefs and western public health methods. This particular combination was favoured by the rise of a cultural current known as indigenism, which stimulated a positive reappraisal of Indian beliefs and eased the introduction of new health practices. The leading actor in this story was Manuel Núñez Butrón, a physician who organized a health brigade and published a medical journal for the people. The work done by Núñez Butrón respected communitarian values and simultaneously used the Indian people to extend smallpox vaccination and promote a campaign against epidemic typhus.

Puno

Núñez Butrón worked in the *altiplano* of Puno, an enormous expanse of land located on the shores of Lake Titicaca at more than 3800 metres above sea level, which has a harsh, cold and dry climate. The *altiplano* has been inhabited by two distinct linguistic groups since pre-Columbian times: the Quechua and the Aymara. In the nineteenth century the city of Puno, on the shores of Lake Titicaca, was the commercial and administrative centre of the region. Trade carried out by boat connected the city with the towns around the lake in Peru and Bolivia. Puno was one of the most miserable, marginal and backward departments of Peru until the late nineteenth century.[1] However, Puno began to change in the early twentieth century due to the expansion of the Andean camelid wool trade, and to cattle and sheep raising. Most of the wool was exported to Europe. The Indian population used it only in handcrafts like hats, ponchos and gloves. Although it never attained the importance of other exports like sugar and copper, by 1918 wool had become the second export item in terms of the revenue accruing to the government.[2] The destination of the Puno wool trade was the port of Mollendo in Arequipa, from whence it was exported to the rest of the world.

Puno increased its contacts with the outside world thanks to the wool trade, and lost part of its isolation. A railway line joining Arequipa and Cuzco via the department of Puno was completed in 1908. What matters here is that the railway went to the new and more accessible city of Juliaca, some 47 kilometres from the city of Puno. Juliaca became from then on a crucial centre for goods going into and out of the *altiplano*.[3] This entailed the decline of the old city of Puno, but it nonetheless retained its administrative role as departmental capital. The sudden rise in importance of Juliaca attracted a small community of white and blue collar workers, and merchants, including a group of Italians who sold groceries, gave credit to the *haciendas* and took part in the wool trade. This city, which was going through a modernizing process right in the middle of a traditional Indian area, was the headquarters of Núñez Butrón.

Most of the peasants in Puno lived in communities with a long history, controlled their land, sold their produce and had a high degree of political autonomy. The communities coexisted side by side with great landed estates which were in the hands of no more than a few individuals, just like in other parts of southern Peru. The favourable conditions present in the wool market made many landowners expand their holdings at the expense of the communal lands. Some Indian holdings were literally assaulted and absorbed by the great *haciendas*. This sparked off a series of Indian revolts between 1900 and 1920. The most famous of these was the revolt led in 1915 by Sergeant Teodomiro Gutiérrez Cuevas, alias 'Rumi Maqui', who demanded the return of the land to the peasants and the restoration of Tawantinsuyu, the old Inca empire.[4] These revolts were put down by force with the help of the gendarmerie and the army.

The conflict between landowners and Indian communities decreased after 1925.[5] This was partly because of the fall in the international demand for Peruvian wool. The discovery of new synthetic fibres, the preference England had for its colonial possessions after the First World War and, later, the world crisis of 1930 all affected the demand for Puno wool. The other factor behind the easing of conflict was the successful resistance of the Indian communities, which prevented the loss of all their land. A relative social peace was established in the region in the late 1920s, which was not due to the defeat of Indian organizations but to an economic recession, and to the political stalemate between *hacendados* and Indian communities. Social tension therefore fell and legal and non-violent methods became the preferred channels of dealing with conflicts. The sanitary brigade organized by Núñez Butrón carried out its activities in this context, which emphasized co-operation instead of confrontation. The new political spirit favoured the brigade because it received the support of different groups including landowners, merchants and peasant organizations for a common goal: public health. The peaceful social conditions likewise allowed the communities to provide resources and volunteers.

Another characteristic of this region that stimulated the rise of the brigade was Adventism and its interest in hygiene. North American and Argentinian Seventh Day Adventist pastors were in the *altiplano* since 1909. Adventist pastors visited the Indian towns acting as physicians and teachers, but only stayed where their services were requested. The Adventists were greeted first out of curiosity, and then with sympathy in several remote areas where neither state nor church, schools or western medicine were known. By 1919 they had established an important preaching centre in Platería.

One of the goals the Adventists had was to change some pernicious Indian customs like the abuse of alcohol and coca leaves. The habit of chewing coca had religious and cultural origins, and was caused by the stress of manual labour. Coca allayed hunger and helped forget fatigue, thus partially easing peasant labours. However, it has toxic effects when misused and when the user is in a state of malnutrition. The Adventists boosted the self-esteem of those who embraced their creed. Apparently they were successful. A Limeño writer was startled to find that the Adventist 'Indian' had a quality that was unusual in Andean people: they were proud of who they were: 'he looks you in the eye and greets without kissing the hand ... he is aware of his most essential rights and duties'.[6] The Adventists were harassed by the Bishop of Puno, but in 1915 the National Congress eliminated the restrictions curtailing the celebration of public ceremonies for non-Catholics. An index of their influence is that in 1916 there were 19 Adventist elementary schools in Puno, but by 1926 their number had risen to 80. According to the 1940 census, Puno was by far the Peruvian department with the most Protestants.[7]

Many of the leaders of the Indian sanitary brigade were Adventists, and later co-operated with Núñez Butrón. Besides, some felt their participation in the brigade was an extension of their religious activities. According to Melchor Cutipa Coaquira, an Adventist who worked with Núñez Butrón, the work of the brigade was part of his religious activities.[8] Although a Catholic, Núñez Butrón trusted the Adventists because he found in them volunteers who were used to sacrificing themselves for their communities, had received an elementary education and were able to communicate in public.

Concern over rural education was not monopolized by the Adventists. The distance between Puno and the decision centres made the official educational system neglect the department. According to a national educational census carried out in 1902, only 11 per cent of the boys in the department between 4 and 14 years of age received any education.[9] A group of provincial intellectuals tried to change this by promoting Indian education. The most renowned of them was the educator José Antonio Encinas, who directed an elementary school in Puno from 1906 to 1911, where indigenous languages were taught.[10] Some of his students who became teachers in their own communities backed the activities of Núñez Butrón, and expanded the brigade's goals by establishing elementary schools where lessons on hygiene had an important place.

The work of Encinas and the sanitary activities of Núñez Butrón were part of the rise of a regional and ethnic nationalist movement in provincial Peru known as *indigenismo*.[11] Lima and some Andean cities had been undergoing an intense process of cultural renewal since the turn of the century, which expressed itself in the development of intellectual currents that sought to change the negative image of Indians then prevalent in society. Indigenism developed as a literary movement that idealized the Inca empire. This new current was taken to Lima by writers, journalists and university students from the provinces who rejected the positivist trend that held Indians as an inferior race which arrested development, or as minors fit only for handcrafts, the army and servitude. For these intellectuals, Indian society, history and culture had to be reappraised if the natives were to be integrated.[12]

Indigenism was also construed as the development of a new national identity whose focus would be the pre-Columbian culture that had survived centuries of hardships. Its mildest variant rejected racism, ignored the economic aspects of Indian exploitation and sponsored beneficial laws like the universalization of elementary education or universal conscription. In its most radical variants, indigenism was a reverse racism, or proposed the elimination of the *haciendas*. Although indigenism had its roots in literature, its influence extended to politics, painting, the social sciences and medicine.[13]

Indigenism was eclipsed among Lima's intellectuals in the late 1930s, and was replaced by hispanism. This current entailed a derogatory appraisal of pre-Columbian culture, and an overemphasis on Peru's Hispanic heritage. Spurred by the Spanish Civil War and the subsequent victory of Franco, conservative intellectuals emphasized Hispanic traditions and rejected the idealization of the Andean world. Conditions were different in the South Andean cities, where indigenism developed before the 1920s and remained active until the early 1940s. Some examples of these developments were the rise of cultural societies like Bohemia Andina, Orkopatta and Laykakota in Puno, and journals like *Kosko*, *La Sierra*, *Kuntur* and the *Boletín Titikaka*.[14] These organizations and journals were a proud vindication of the culture and history of provincial Peru which criticized Lima's centralism, and outlined the identity of Andean intellectuals. For Valcárcel, a trait that distinguished Puno's *indigenistas* was their great involvement with social movements: some even took part in preparing the demands of peasant uprisings.[15] One example of this kind of intellectual was Rodríguez Aweranka, who belonged to the Orkopatta group, was educated by Encinas, and later on collaborated with Núñez Butrón. Both Rodríguez Aweranka and Núñez Butrón were influenced in their youth by Indian movements and by the *indigenistas*. We will consider below their sanitation activities as part of a full-scale vindication of Indian culture and society. The other leaders of Núñez Butron's brigade also lived in a cultural environment marked by indigenism, whether they were Catholics or Adventists.

In brief, three factors explain the context in which the sanitary work of Núñez Butrón took place: the relative social peace established between Indian communities and the great landed estates (which made it possible to derive resources from several sources); the promotion of hygiene and education by the Adventists (which prepared Indian leaders ready to work for their own communities); and the spread of indigenism among provincial intellectuals (thus creating a favourable feeling for Indian culture).

Núñez Butrón

Some aspects in the biography of Núñez Butrón are also useful to understand the Indian sanitary brigade he led. Manuel Núñez Butrón was born in 1899 in Samán, a small town in the southern corner of the province of Azángaro. He was the acknowledged illegitimate child of a Catholic priest and a middle-class mestizo woman.[16] His case was not uncommon in the Andes, for it was usual for illegitimate children to be recognized. In his early years, Núñez Butrón faced the obstacles, pressures and expectations for social mobility that surely characterized the life of the few young Puneños who could get a formal education.[17] When he was 17, Núñez Butrón wrote an impassioned article in a school paper that showed his desire to be outstanding in his work, and his concern for social justice:

> not to live just for the sake of it. To live for coming generations, not as a parasite ... work is essential to repair our umpteen needs ... our sensibility, our intelligence and our will shall pass away, but their deeds will be perpetuated in time ... What is left for Peruvians, after seeing how ambition seeks to prevail over justice? Nothing but work, work and work, turning the present into a future.[18]

In an autobiographical statement, Núñez Butrón would later tell how throughout his studies he had trouble with his identity over being called an Indian or a *misti* (the Spanish name given to whites living in the Andes).[19] It was not just a racial difference. *Mistis* spoke Spanish, were literate, lived in cities, and usually belonged to the middle and upper classes. In his home town, Núñez Butrón was considered a *misti* because his parents spoke Spanish. He was later considered an Indian while attending elementary school in Juliaca because he came from inside the province. Núñez Butrón managed to be held on equal footing with the rest of his classmates after some years of effort, congeniality and skill. The same experience happened all over again when he went to study in the renowned San Carlos school in Puno – the only high school in the department since 1851 – where no one wanted to accept him as a *misti* because he came from Juliaca, which was considered a less important town.

Teenagers from families living beside the lake were of no disposition to accept a boy from Samán, or even Juliaca, as one of their peers. Núñez Butrón once again managed to assert himself and be accepted by his schoolmates. The clash was probably stronger when he went to study science in the University of San Agustín in Arequipa, and the cycle of rejection and acceptance was repeated once more. Arequipa, the second city in Peru in terms of its population and trade, was the favourite abode for many immigrant families of European origin, and had a white and mestizo elite which was more clearly removed from the rest of society. For this elite, the path to upward mobility was closed by rigid racial, cultural and economic criteria.

Núñez Butrón told with some resentment how Arequipa's university students would shout 'Indian' at him in the street, as if it were a great insult. The act of living together, the debates, sports and perhaps some fistfights, won him the appreciation of the locals. Finally, the same story of an initial rejection due to racial and geographic reasons and his eventual acceptance for cultural and personal qualities was repeated once more in Lima, where he studied in San Marcos University for one year. It is worth pointing out that when he enrolled in San Marcos he registered as a native of Arequipa, either because it was a habit of the Puneño students, or because his birth certificate was registered in Yanahuara, Arequipa.[20] Then he returned to the city of Puno in one of his vacations and felt somewhat superior because no one could now call him an Indian. We can well imagine that for a young Puneño, being an alumnus of San Marcos was a status symbol. It is also proof that although Peruvian education was not a road to upward social mobility for all young men from the provinces, it was so indeed for some accomplished individuals like him.

However, this was not to be the end to his identity problems. Núñez Butrón travelled to Spain to study medicine in Barcelona, enticed by the chance to study in Europe and the temporary closure of San Marcos in 1921, due to a strike among the professors.[21] In Spain, all of his long, previous efforts were not enough for him to achieve a new victory on the same scale as his previous ones. In spite of speaking the same language he was always called an Indian just because he came from Peru. According to Núnez Butrón, his Spanish classmates did not care whether he was from Juliaca, Arequipa or Lima: they could not perceive the subtle differences between an Indian and a *misti* (a term which was valid only in Peru). They simply identified him as Peruvian, that is, an Indian.

The consistent response of the Spaniards left an indelible mark on the personality of Núñez Butrón. For him, 'those who were not Indians' made him become 'fond of the Indians'. It was only then that he realized that the 'previous transformations were of customs, not of race', and began to identify himself with his Indian cultural heritage.[22] It was only in Barcelona that indigenism finally crystallized his own identity. However, this only showed on his return to Peru in 1925.

The experience of Núñez Butrón in Barcelona during 1921–25 was also important for other reasons. The culture, university and medicine in this city were then undergoing a twin process of Europeanization and nationalism. This process showed in a closeness to European science, particularly with the experimental tradition of French physiology, and the retrieval of Catalan as a valid language for academic events and specialized journals. The teachers of Núñez Butrón included leaders of Spanish medicine like Augusto Pi Suñer, the President of the Biological Society of Barcelona, and Andrés Martínez Vargas, the founder of the Spanish Pediatric Society. His best marks (outstanding and distinguished) were in anatomy, physiology and pathology. (He just 'passed' in 'hygiene with bacteriological practices'.) Spanish sanitation was likewise undergoing a process of renewal which showed in the organization of sanitary brigades and popularizing campaigns.[23]

Núñez Butrón returned to Peru in 1925 and briefly entertained the idea of settling down in Lima.[24] His foreign degree would certainly have attracted clients. However, after working for some months in Lima in a school and as a military medic, Núñez Butrón returned to Puno where he was successively appointed state physician in the provinces of Azángaro, Huancané, Lampa and San Román.

Health in Puno

By the late 1920s, the department of Puno was one of the poorest areas in Peru, and one of the most neglected by the State. The 1940 census indicates a high correlation between illiteracy, overcrowding and lack of water and sanitary facilities.[25]

The miserable living conditions and the government's neglect had made typhoid fever, dysentery and other diseases endemic, particularly smallpox and epidemic typhus. Some had existed since the colonial period and had been given several Quechua names, like *muru* for smallpox and *hatun onkoy* (the great disease), *tabardillo* and *tuila* for typhus.[26] For most Puneños, these diseases were caused by supernatural forces unleashed by deities, by enemies and by not observing rituals like paying homage to the ancestors, the earth and other elements of nature. In Puno, the Indians believed health depended on a harmonious and grateful relationship with some sacred mountains where the *achachilas*, or guardian spirits of the community who looked after the welfare of people, plants and animals, lived. In Chucuito (Puno), the power to divine the unknown, cure diseases and coax the spirits was shared by several individuals such as the *paccos* (seers), *laiccas* (witches), *colasiri* (healers), *yatiris* (fortune-tellers), *coliris* (nurses) and *usuriris* (midwives). Each of these practitioners had different roles, but what was usually asked of them was to uncover ecological and social imbalances or the behaviour that had caused the disease, and re-establish the balance between the patient, the community and the environment.[27]

In order to understand why epidemic typhus and smallpox were endemic in the Andes and less frequent on the coast we need to point out some characteristics of these diseases. Epidemic typhus is caused by a micro-organism (*Rickettsia prowazekii*) which, like all *Rickettsias*, is halfway between viruses and bacteria, and is only transmitted from a sick person to a healthy one by the *Pediculus humanus* louse, which lives close to the warmth of the human body, in the hair and in clothes.[28] It is important to point out that overcrowding, unhygienic conditions and low temperatures are the environmental conditions that create a favourable environment for epidemic typhus, a disease characterized by a high fever, prostration, headaches, body aches and a rash all over the body. In Puno, the harshness of the weather, the lack of fuel and poverty, as shown by the possession of just one ragged dress, all helped the disease spread. Places like army barracks, jails and the overcrowded huts of Andean Indians provided the essential conditions for the spread of typhus. These dwellings had only one small, dark and constricted room built of adobe bricks and straw, with an earthen floor and without any light or ventilation. The dwellers slept on the floor or on adobe platforms, wrapped in dirty rags and shorn leather. According to one witness, in an Indian dwelling in Puno lived 'the family with the children and next of kin, and where they sleep they eat, cook, store their provisions and household goods'.[29]

The disease also spread thanks to peasants travelling to country fairs and to work as seasonal labourers in the countryside. The wool trade entailed the decline of the natural economy and the replacement of annual fairs with more frequent ones. Lice spread the disease through the crowds of people who went to the markets and religious ceremonies, and there was also contagion due to some Andean customs such as watching over the dead for several days, sleeping in the same bed with the sick, and washing the deceased's clothes eight days later. In some parts of the highlands it was believed that children should not have their hair cut between birth and their second birthday (when a special ceremony took place) because doing so to the newly born weakened their teeth.[30]

The areas most affected by epidemic typhus were the central and southern cordilleras of Peru. The low temperatures and scant humidity in these areas located at more than 2000 metres above sea level favoured the spread of *Rickettsia*. The coast and the Amazon forest were free of epidemic typhus.[31] At the turn of the twentieth century, Peruvian physicians believed typhus was a highland disease due to a combination of climatic factors, such as temperature, biological factors, like the immunity produced by the disease, and social factors, like the overcrowded dwellings of Andean peasants.[32] A study made in the 1920s noted that 'typhus is not contagious where the temperature is over 20 degrees [and even more so] on the coast ... the disease has never appeared [there]'. This distribution made a physician prepare a map of the disease:

> If we wanted to represent the extent and number of cases of epidemic typhus in surface area and in depth, we would have to picture the typhoid area like a pyramid resting on the Andes, with its rectangular base on the departments of the southern highlands, and decreasing in scope and incidence as we move to the Andean departments in the northern part of the country.[33]

The persistence of the disease's magnitude is reflected by the testimony of a subprefect in Puno who complained in the early nineteenth century that epidemic typhus took a great toll and whittled down communities 'with more than two hundred Indians ... to eight or ten families'. The years for which reliable statistics exist show the greater prevalence of the disease in the highlands. For instance, in 1950 the mortality rate of typhus in the highlands was 100 cases per 100 000 inhabitants, while it was no more than 31 cases in the coastlands. In the Amazon forest it was just 1 per 100 000 inhabitants.[34] An indirect and inefficient way of controlling epidemic typhus was the habit of delousing people manually and then chewing the lice. According to Indian beliefs, this practice bestowed immunity, and a certain amount of lice were needed by the body because 'they took bad blood away'.[35] Urine was likewise used to wash the hair because it was believed it 'removed the filth'.[36] Furthermore, according to a physician in Cuzco 'decomposing urine [*pocko-jispay*]' was commonly used 'as a panacea, to be taken either pure or with salt, or to be used to treat several ailments'.[37]

Around 1930, the only way of controlling the disease was by eliminating the lice and keeping a good personal hygiene, shaving one's hair and using clean clothes. However, not even this was done. In the introductory clauses of a 1931 bill it was acknowledged that as far as typhus was concerned, there 'never has been ... a well organized campaign'.[38] It was not until the 1950s that an effective combination of a vaccine and an insecticide appeared. When Núñez Butrón was alive, controlling typhus entailed a disciplined organization that promoted hygiene.

The other prominent disease in the highlands against which the brigade fought was smallpox, from which Núñez Butrón himself had suffered, and which left its scars on his face. *Variola major*, the deadliest variety of the disease, was much feared in the Andes since the colonial period due to its high mortality and its sequels: disfigurement, blindness and incapacitation. Smallpox was produced by a virus directly transmitted from one person to another, mainly through drops of saliva from the nose or the mouth. (This requires closeness, a common occurrence in the overcrowded living conditions of the Andes.) The disease usually began with a high fever, a violent cold, a headache and pain in the waist and back, plus a strange difficulty in looking at lights.[39] Later, pimples appeared on the skin, particularly on the face and limbs, which itched terribly and became pustules. Finally, some yellow scabs appeared which on falling left pockmarks behind for life.

Smallpox was a disease without any cure; it killed or bequeathed permanent immunity. Those who survived had their face pocked with small marks, which is why on the coast they were known as *borrados* (erased) and *cacaruñados* (damaged face) and *fieros* (fierce) in the highlands. In the Andes they were believed to be the strongest and were preferred for marriage, as they warranted immunity in the face of one of the most feared diseases.[40] The absence of any stigma was due to the extent of the disease. There was some stoicism in the face of smallpox, and even epidemic typhus, which led to their being accepted as an everyday, unavoidable event. This is also borne out by the Indian belief that smallpox was caused by an errant, capricious and evil deity who attacked without warning. It was believed that this being kept watch from a corner in the room when visitors came to see the sick, and got upset when the bedclothes were shaken, when people cried in front of the deceased or when his name was mentioned. One was advised to pay homage to the deity with flowers and fruits to ease its wrath, take children to the house of the sick in order that the deity would recognize them and to pick up the clothes of the deceased eight days after its burial.[41]

Vaccination was the only efficient prevention method known since 1798, when it was popularized by Edward Jenner. In Peru, vaccination arrived in 1804 with a Spanish expedition and was promoted in a limited fashion during the nineteenth century, first through the parish priests and then the municipalities, which created the post of 'Inspector of Hygiene and Vaccines' in the late nineteenth century.[42] Things improved somewhat in 1896 when vaccination became compulsory, a specialized institution was established (the National [Institute] of Vaccines and Serotherapy), and the government created the post of Vaccinator (1905). The enforcement of the law remained in the hands of the municipalities, and vaccination was carried out in plazas and markets. In 1908, regulations established a fine for parents, tutors or employers who resisted the vaccination of their children and employees. The measure was not fully enforced, because in 1928 the executive power had to take over vaccination. Besides the resistance shown by the people, there also was the problem of keeping the vaccines refrigerated.[43] In Puno, healers and many others mistrusted the vaccine for several reasons. They believed it could transmit smallpox and other diseases like syphilis (which was true) and some feared that the vaccination records were used to establish new taxes. Healers preferred to prevent the disease by ingesting scabs of those sick with smallpox, and used a juice prepared with cow dung as medicine.[44]

Smallpox declined on the coast and in all major cities after the 1920s due to a greater distribution of vaccines. By 1919 this lowered the cases of smallpox in parts of the northern highlands like Cajamarca.[45] In the south, the long distances and unstable transportation systems often meant that the vaccines sent from Lima arrived in useless condition. Besides, in Andean populations 'the resistance [of the people] is greater, and the help of the police is sometimes needed'.[46]

It was only in 1943 that the Ministry of Health established the National Vaccination Service, in response to a brutal epidemic of smallpox that had ravaged Ayacucho. The Service widened its scope and the number of people vaccinated rose from 339 603 in 1940 to 1 876 406 in 1944. With the support of the Pan American Health Bureau, smallpox declined from 3600 cases in 1950 to zero in 1955. It reappeared in 1964, and a campaign based on a cheaper vaccine that was applied to 5.5 million people had completely eradicated the disease from Peru by 1967. Shortly after, the disease was eradicated throughout the world.[47]

In Puno in the 1930s, the problem in carrying out vaccination lay in getting the support of Lima, in overcoming the resistance of the population and in finding a group of vaccinators. Núñez Butrón had few resources with which to begin this task. According to the 1940 census, in the department there were just 26 individuals specialized in the health professions, i.e. doctors, nurses, technicians and obstetricians which, for a population of 646 385 gave a mean of 24 860 inhabitants for each professional. This was even more serious if we bear in mind that 92 per cent of the population was scattered throughout the countryside.[48]

In Lima, where more than half the health professionals of Peru worked, the mean in 1940 was of one per 362 inhabitants. According to this same census, the national mean was of 2224 inhabitants for each professional. According to a 1930 report, 3775 beds out of the 5213 in 44 hospitals were on the coast, 1373 in the highlands and 65 in the Amazon forest.[49]

The lack of physicians in the provinces was due to the low salaries paid to state physicians, the instability of the appointments due to the non-existence of a state-sponsored health career (it was only in 1937 that health became a part of the civil service), the lack of clients who could support a professional practice, and the costs in terms of transportation and communications incurred by a roving physician. The duties of state physicians included free assistance in hospitals, morgues, jails, army barracks and public offices. On the other hand, physicians had few colleagues with whom they could interact and had to depend on the whims of the authorities when it came to obtaining resources.[50] Working in the provinces was therefore lonely and daunting.

Although the law forced state physicians to live in provincial capitals, most preferred to live in the capital city of the department. In a country where medicine was a professional occupation only in cities, young physicians avoided settling in remote areas. The School of Medicine of San Marcos had an urban and clinical orientation, with little emphasis on research and public health.[51]

A quote from Núñez Butrón illustrates the hardships a state physician had to endure in the Peruvian Andes:

> The government pays the State physician ... to fight the epidemics which break out in his jurisdiction, but what can a man do, no matter how good a scientist he is, if his duty it is to look after thousands of people scattered hundreds of kilometres around? What can a young, newly graduated physician from medical school do, if he only has one thermometer and a prescription book? The thermometer will not last long, and the prescription book is useful to prescribe drugs which will arrive after several days have gone by, long after the sick person has died.[52]

In these conditions, many provincial physicians only looked after the sick who lived in the countryside when an epidemic broke out, or when they had some spare time. Their activities were concentrated in urban centres where they looked after the middle and upper classes, and where they could earn money on the side by selling medicines to their patients or managing a pharmacy.[53]

Núñez Butrón tried to go beyond the traditional role of provincial physicians. Since most of the sick could not go to Juliaca, he decided to travel to different locations first on horseback, then on a motorcycle and, finally, by car. He soon realized this method was inadequate and that he needed assistants. In his travels he established contact with people who were ready to co-operate, and then organized them in a brigade.

The sanitary brigade

In 1933, Núñez Butrón established the first sanitary brigade in Isla, a community with a population of slightly over 31 000 near Juliaca.[54] The brigade and its members were given the Quechua name of *rijchary*, which translates as 'awaken'. The name had a deep, ethnic connotation. The notion of awakening the Indian race had been previously mentioned by the indigenists, and suggested that the backwardness of the native groups was not a permanent condition.[55] Each *rijchary* received an armband from the Red Cross (even though there was no formal connection with it) and a document recording his appointment. An article in the journal that the brigade published shows an idealized account of the dedication and ascetism of the *rijcharys*: 'they speak the languages [Quechua and Aymara] ... do not look for places to entertain themselves in ... They live with their people ... They are not sanitarians to cure but *rijcharys* to prevent'.[56] New brigades appeared later in Rancho, Chacas and Collana, and in other communities.

The leaders of the first brigade were the Cutipa Coaquira brothers, Adventists who had finished elementary school. Some Indians who had served in the army for two years were also members of the brigade. It is worth pointing out that those Indians who returned to their communities after their military experience (which usually entailed moving to an urban area) had been exposed to new cultural patterns and now became natural local leaders. For instance, Eustakio Rodríguez Aweranka was a former soldier who became one of the prominent figures of the brigade. (An additional qualification was that he was fluent in Spanish, Quechua and Aymara.) Lastly, the brigade included healers and herbalists who accepted some of Núñez Butrón's methods without fully abandoning their beliefs. According to a brigade leader, instead of persecuting the healers these were sought to 'praise their labours in areas where medicine would never arrive … [and so] take advantage of their suggestive powers … [and] preempt the campaign they could have organized against medicine'.[57] Núñez Butrón occasionally resorted to magical explanations to recommend the anti-smallpox vaccine as a medicine against 'all evils', and he himself used herbs and poultices (a technique from traditional medicine) to heal injuries.[58]

The recruitment of Adventists, former soldiers and healers widened the acceptance of Núñez Butrón's sanitary discourse, and stimulated the Indian communities to look after their own health. Instead of blindly relying on the presumed supremacy of western medicine, he legitimized his activities through his connection with the natural leaders of the communities. It was a different attitude from that of others who were in charge of public health, and who considered that this was an exclusively technical matter which was hindered by traditional medicine and the ignorance of the people. The complaints made in 1939 by an official of the Ministry of Health are therefore illustrative: 'The Indian … frankly or craftily opposes the performance of the authorities … [he] rebels against all innovation … [and] goes so far as to destroy what science creates precisely for him.'[59]

Although this was the most common attitude among physicians, it is worth pointing out that the officials in the military regime that ruled Peru in the 1930s did give some formal support to Núñez Butrón. Proof of this is the establishment, in 1936, during the administration of General Óscar Benavides, of health brigades to reinforce the work done by state physicians, particularly in cases of epidemics. Apparently these brigades did not function, but their establishment indicates that Núñez Butrón had the support of officials in Lima.[60] This enabled him to divide the salary meant for an assistant between four members of the brigade. The help given by the highest authority in the province of San Román to several meetings of the brigade is also indicative of official support locally.

To prevent epidemic typhus, the brigades concentrated on vaccination and the promotion of hygiene. They also assisted at childbirths, gave injections, cut hair, deloused people, supplied aspirin, gave purgatives, disinfected rooms, pulled out teeth, taught how to make soup and built small stoves which killed the fleas without damaging the clothes.[61] The brigade members worked first in their own communities and then in neighbouring ones, as if they were itinerant doctors. In doing so they were repeating the traditional way of practising medicine in the southern Andes. The quacks and the renowned herbalists of Kallawaya, in Bolivia, travelled throughout the south Andes, offering their medicines and herbs.[62] The members of the brigade also made themselves known at fairs and Sunday markets held in Juliaca and other urban centres, where goods were sold or bartered.

In a typical day's work, the brigade called the people to the town square. In the assembly, its members presented in simple fashion the advantages posed by hygiene and vaccination. For instance, they used a poster with a louse, showed a clean and a dirty child, and sang folk songs with the lyrics altered to promote nationalism, literacy and hygiene. The assembly included a lecture by Núñez Butrón or Rodríguez Aweranka. Once the lecture was over, the crowd was inoculated with the anti-smallpox vaccine, given haircuts and bathed in the river. (This resembled the Adventist ritual of baptism.) The cultural programme of the brigade was enhanced when the *rijcharys* began to celebrate 24 June as Indian Day with marathon races, dances, speeches, hygiene exhibitions and a parade through the streets of Juliaca. The celebration, in which no alcohol was taken, ended with a general assembly on the Huayna Roque, the hill over the city, and soap, books, scissors and pencils provided by local merchants were distributed.[63]

Apparently, the rise in the number of activities carried out by the brigade went hand in hand with a decrease in the importance of traditional healers. The influence of the Kallawaya herbalists and other native practitioners began to decline after the 1930s, and doctors and pharmacists began to go to the Andes in greater numbers.[64] These often felt the healers were their competitors, and should be denounced and held in check. Pharmaceutical companies, mainly of Peruvian and German origin, began to expand in the country advertising manufactured medicines and biological products. On the other hand, the economic modernization which Juliaca was going through influenced part of the population and made it reject what it considered traditional, like Indian medicine.

A decisive step in the development of the brigades was the publication, in April 1935, of the journal *Runa Soncco*. According to its publishers, in Quechua this meant 'Indian heart' or 'he who loves the Indian with all his heart'.[65] Funds for the journal were obtained through Núñez Butrón himself, some subscriptions, and the co-operation of some friends. In its first issue, the journal defined itself as a publication by 'the Indians for the Indians'.[66] The effectiveness of a journal can be doubted in a society that was mostly illiterate. According to the 1940 census, only 14 per cent of the people in the department were literate.[67] However, some testimonies assert that the journal was read out loud by a member of the brigade.

Although epidemic typhus and smallpox always received most attention in the journal, some articles dealt with other common diseases like syphilis and tuberculosis. The journal criticized habits that favoured typhus but without belittling them, such as not cutting children's hair or placing them in the bed of someone sick with smallpox. (This was done because it was believed that it was better for the infection to take place at an age when the children have possibilities of surviving the disease.) Another popular habit discussed in the journal was *pichaska*, or bathing the sick with cow's milk, which was then sold in the market in the belief that this procedure soothed the pain of the pustules, and that the purchaser bought the disease. A similar custom had people preparing a bundle with the clothes of the sick person, and leaving them on the road for someone to pick up.[68]

An article in *Runa Soncco* approved and compared the advantages of some home methods employed by the Indians to control lice, such as the use of nitrous earth (*kallpa*), leaving wet clothes outside so the cold would kill the lice (*kasacheska*), placing clothes in containers with boiling water (*putesca*) or eating hot peppers, parsley or cumin. The journal even found a rationale for the use of urine when washing the hair, in the amount of ammonia that urine has.[69] Around the 1940s, Núñez Butrón described the attitude shown by the members of the brigade saying that they first studied the psychology of the people. It was only 'when they have managed to convince them with their own ideas, [that] those in need come in search of science'. For Núñez Butrón, understanding folk medicine was not just a matter of sanitation pedagogy; it was essential to develop sanitarian activities adapted to local conditions: 'the Altimampino and the scientific methods are almost the same, and are only distinguished by the degree of their effects'.[70] *Runa Soncco* also described debating sessions between the *rijcharys* and peasants on the magical origins of smallpox. Once, after the *rijcharys* convinced their rivals of the bacterial origins of the disease and the advantages of vaccination, all ended the meeting shouting 'Three cheers for Jenner even though he is dead!'[71]

Only ten issues of *Runa Soncco* were published during 1935–48, six of them between 1935 and 1937. The latter were the most significant years of the *rijcharys*. In 1937 the brigade comprised 122 members who looked after 22 different localities, from whence they had to send reports periodically. Fourteen of these were Indian communities located in the Quechua area around Lake Titicaca, and belonged to the provinces of Azángaro, San Román, Lampa and Huancané, which had a total population of 189 000 according to the 1940 census.[72]

In the first six months of 1937, the *rijcharys* carried out 10 000 vaccinations and cut the hair of slightly over 600 people. Besides, Núñez Butrón built the first hospital in Juliaca where the headquarters of the brigade had once been. An itinerant library and at least 12 schools directly connected with the organization were built under the slogan 'we want to continue being Indians, but with a library in our heads'. Some arithmetic lessons published in *Runa Soncco* contributed to the work of these schools.[73] The brigade paid attention to problems closely connected to health such as education, and thus promoted a process of integrated social development. *Runa Soncco* did not limit itself to articles on sanitation, but dealt with everyday events like birthdays, baptisms, deaths, weddings and *servinacuys* (the variable amount of time a betrothed couple lived together, after which they married). The journal also included descriptions of local customs, riddles and poems. Reference was usually made to the subject of health. One of the first translations of the national anthem into Quechua and Aymara, which was done by Rodríguez Aweranka, was published on the cover of the journal.[74]

Runa Soncco reflected the desire to integrate Andean culture and western public health. A medical publication of this kind cannot be understood without bearing in mind the context of the indigenist movement. Some articles in *Runa Soncco* clearly reveal the indigenism of their authors. One addressed to 'the Indians' asserted that a change of behaviour was an act of racial and personal vindication: 'Are you not human just because you are an Indian? ... do not cast away your humanity. Wash your body and clean your clothing.'[75] The document certifying the appointment of the *rijcharys* included some pointers like: 'impart the pride of being an Indian'.[76] Some parts of the journal carried suggestive and proud mottos such as 'To disavow one's race indicates ignorance'.[77]

Indigenism had usually been a literary, artistic and political movement, but in Puno it appeared as medical indigenism. The brigade organized by Núñez Butrón was a movement inspired by the belief that the salvation of the Indian race lay not just in passing favourable bills, possessing land and recovering their culture, but also in its mastery of hygiene and education. Furthermore, according to one article the major problem for the Indian was 'the health problem'.[78] The leaders of the brigade praised the inborn ability of the Indian race to create a clean environment and change habits which favoured the development of diseases. This medical indigenism could not avoid being influenced by political ideas, and as a result its members began to inquire about the social basis of disease in the Andes.

Health and society

It is important to point out that the political tone of the journal was at first moderate. For instance, a 1937 editorial stated that 'after so many centuries it is hard to set a dividing line between the conquered and the conquerors. One way or the other, before the world we all are INDIANS'.[79] However, some articles in *Runa Soncco* moved well beyond a timid indigenism or the promotion of hygiene, and invaded the world of social critique to probe the ultimate causes of disease. The members of the brigade not only campaigned against alcoholism and coca-chewing (like the Adventists) but also criticized the merchants who promoted coca and alcohol consumption. The articles bitterly attacked lawyers, true and false, and the so-called 'lawsuit-mania'. This referred to the proclivity Indians had of going to court to solve the disputes between Indians, and between their communities and the rural estates (*haciendas*). Since the Indians usually lacked legally acceptable titles, the *hacendados* could take the land from the communities with impunity under the protection of the local judges.[80]

A 1937 issue of *Runa Soncco* showed that an indigenist-inspired social critique could combine racial and hygienic criteria. One motto suggestively read: 'lice are the *gamonales*[81] who cause the highest number of dead among us'. Another article drew a metaphor in openly racial terms: 'If there are Indians and Cholos who are dirty and have lice on their bodies, there are more than a few whiteys who have lice and filth in their spirit ... Peru owes many of its misfortunes to this kind of dirt.'[82] This kind of critique and the ethnic, autonomous and popular undertones the brigade assumed, aroused the suspicion of the regional power groups. The Church was suspicious of the active co-operation of the Adventists, the merchants were annoyed due to the campaigns against alcohol, lawyers felt themselves attacked because of the critiques made against 'lawsuit-mania' and the *hacendados* were afraid that educating the Indians would make them more skilled in upholding their rights. The time came when the subprefect of Juliaca prohibited the opening of a new *rijchary* school in Isla, and an orderly parade of the brigade members through the streets of Juliaca upset the enemies of Núñez Butrón.[83] As a result, the pressures to decapitate the movement mounted and Núñez Butrón was transferred to the Amazonian province of Ucayali in 1937. He was there for just a few months, when in mid-1938 he was transferred as state physician to the province of Angaraes in Huancavelica.[84] This kind of semi-exile was regarded as punishment by the brigade members.

Little is known of the brigade after 1939, when Núñez Butrón returned to Puno.[85] He probably chose to keep a low profile to avoid trouble. The brigade's scope was reduced to Juliaca and some neighbouring towns. *Runa Soncco* was published erratically between 1945 and 1948, and this shows the brigade did continue some of its activities. However, the tone of the articles hints at decline, resentment and nostalgia: 'There is no doubt that lice, alcohol, and lawsuit-mania have more friends than enemies ... Poor *Runa Soncco* ... It no longer is what it was, but it was what it will be.' There was also a lingering resentment against those who opposed Núñez Butrón: 'I do not know why there is so much opposition to us Indians having a speaker.'[86] An important characteristic of the three issues published from 1945 to 1948 is the inclusion in the subtitle of *Jakke Chuyma*, the Aymara translation of *Runa Soncco*. This suggests a greater identification of Núñez Butrón with Indian culture.

There was more opposition to Núñez Butrón when medical terms were openly used in reference to social ills. One article denounced the survival of feudalism in the province and stated, in regard to Azángaro: 'This town is completely infected with lawsuit-mania. The microbes and bacilli of this social evil: lawyers true and false, pettifoggers ... are a real plague.' The author ended requesting the destruction of the 'pathogenous agent' that gave rise to the ailment of 'lawsuit-mania' and the elimination of its boss, the local landed class.[87]

After this critique, the obvious step in the development of Núñez Butrón was politics. In 1946 he ran for the Chamber of Deputies as representative of the province of San Román. In his campaign, which had health as one of its major subjects, one leaflet gave as his qualities that he had fought epidemics, had opened schools in several hamlets, founded the hospital in Juliaca, and had published *Runa Soncco*, which it defined as a journal inspired by 'a well understood and lofty indigenism'.[88] During the campaign, Núñez Butrón announced his intention to create a vast sanitary movement in southern Peru based on the model of the *rijchary* brigade.

His campaign was backed by several members of the brigade, and by a 'Provincial Committee for the Candidature of Manuel Núñez Butrón'. One of his leaflets said the Constitution ought to be reformed to have 'extremely Peruvian characteristics. Genuinely Andean or *chola* ... an authentic Andean democracy'.[89] However, APRA, the major political force of the time, presented its own candidate and accused Núñez Butrón of having communist support. In the end, Núñez Butron lost the race in a close and questioned result. The campaign raised some charges against the brigade. This was obvious in the 1948 issue of *Runa Soncco*, which bore the following statement on its first page: 'We do not belong to any political party, neither are we financed by anyone. This is just medicine in the service of the Altipampino community.'[90]

The decline of the brigade in the 1940s was also due to cultural factors. Indigenism began its decline in the provinces at the end of this decade, and with it vanished the major cultural backing of Núñez Butrón's activities. The idealization of Indian culture was replaced by the ideologies of modernization that demanded a greater integration in the outside world. The political parties believed that the underdevelopment of the Andean peasantry was the outcome of primitive societies that had to be transformed with limited agrarian reforms and a capitalist exploitation of rural resources.[91] Indigenism was identified with a traditional culture that preserved the status quo and hindered the modernization of rural Peru. Finally, the brigade was greatly dependent on a leader and it declined when its leader lost vigour.

As he grew older, Núñez Butrón began to suffer from chronic mountain sickness, an ailment characterized by the loss of tolerance to altitude in individuals who were previously acclimatized. This condition made him feel tired, gave him headaches, frequently made him feel indisposed and forced him to use oxygen.[92] Besides, he gained weight, which worsened his ailment. Knowing that he would improve if he moved down to sea level, his friends managed to have him appointed to a coastal area, but Núñez Butrón preferred to live in Juliaca and remain close to his family, his friends and his personal belongings. On the other hand, there were rumours that he was chewing coca and drinking heavily. In the late 1940s and early 1950s, Núñez Butrón acquired some of the characteristics of the provincial middle classes. He opened a pharmacy and a medical office in Juliaca, and bought a small site in Arequipa. It was traditional for the Puno middle class to purchase land in Arequipa, as a way of obtaining prestige and security.[93]

During these years Núñez Butrón faced lawsuits which four different women brought against him, claiming support for a total of eight children. The longest of these was begun in 1935 by Lidia Cabrera, his first wife, and ended shortly after his death.[94] Núñez Butrón defended himself stating that in most of the cases he had recognized the children to prevent the mothers from aborting. The 'lawsuit-mania' indicted by *Runa Soncco* as one of the Indians' major problems, was a harsh fact during the last years of its editor.

Manuel Núñez Butrón died in Juliaca in December 1952, when he was only 52. In his will, he requested that an inscription regarding the *rijchary* brigade be placed in his tomb in Arequipa, perhaps because he was well aware that it was the most important achievement of his life.[95] The brigade he created vanished shortly afterwards, but it is worth pointing out that later, the concern over rural medicine was brilliantly taken up again by other physicians in Puno. However, in one of the absurdities with which great stories sometimes end, Eustakio Rodríguez Aweranka migrated to Lima where he earned his living selling pencils on the street.[96]

Conclusion

One of the reasons why the brigade did not survive was the paternalistic role of Núñez Butrón, a role that included authoritarian methods. For instance, he resorted to using the police to force the Indians to bathe in the river and cut their hair, and convinced the head of the Juliaca railway station to demand a certificate of anti-smallpox vaccine from the Indians to whom they sold tickets.[97] Núñez Butrón was able to make these impositions acceptable because he was charismatic. His authority grew because the members of his brigade requested his support to get supplies and to supervise the use of vaccines and medicines. Núñez Butrón was a kind of caudillo whose death left his followers stranded. The institution he created had not been structured to be permanent.

The reception given to *Runa Soncco* throughout Peru was uneven. His work made an impression in the journal *Medicina Social* which was edited in Lima, inspired by the Belgian René Sand, who considered 'social medicine' was an apostolate that patched the deficiencies in official sanitation. Núñez Butrón was aware of this movement, as is suggested by the fact that he was a member of the Argentinian Society for Hygiene and Social Medicine, and that he was recognized during his lifetime by renowned Chilean, Mexican and French physicians who were often members of social medicine organizations.[98] However, the failure to get more support for the activities carried out by Núñez Butrón was not just because Puno was a region far removed from Lima. His work was also different from the main medical trend at the time, which stressed technology and the construction of hospitals. Núñez Butrón gave more importance to hygiene, to intercultural dialogue, to health education and to the transformation of life habits and styles, just like the promoters of primary health care would do years later.

Manuel Núñez Butrón and the brigade he created managed to make western medicine and Indian culture co-operate using few and simple resources. Two factors made this union possible: first, the persistence of indigenism in provincial Peru during the 1930s; second, Núñez Butrón's acquaintance with Indian culture, language and customs. This enabled him to choose the most effective ways of making innovations in their hygiene.

However, the integration of western and Indian culture was never complete. The essential conflict between magical and scientific explanations of disease persisted. Western medicine, even that practised by Núñez Butrón, was still based on the belief that diseases were caused by biological disorders or a malfunctioning organ. For traditional medicine, the roots of the disease lay in an imbalance between the body and the natural, social and religious order where chance, the deities and demons intervened. Núñez Butrón evaded the conflict in an attempt to fuse western therapies and Indian cultural patterns. The magical conception of medicine, which had an empirical basis, accepted these innovations because they did not threaten its overall approach. New lifestyles were accepted because they were useful and could be fitted into the tradition. This compatibility enabled the introduction of haircuts, baths and vaccines, which continued once the brigade left the area.

The sanitary brigade that Núñez Butrón organized managed to create a sanitarian programme that was supported by the Indian communities because it combined self-help with medical paternalism. This experience is still exceptional in Peruvian history. Today, integrating western medicine and Andean cultural patterns remains a difficult task, but as the experience of Manuel Núñez Butrón suggests, it can be done.

Notes

1. Emilio Romero, *Monografía del Departamento de Puno*, Imp. Torres Aguirre, Lima, 1928; Nils Jacobsen, *Mirages of Transition, the Peruvian Altiplano, 1780–1930*, University of California Press, Berkeley, CA, 1993, p. 11.
2. Carlos Barreda, *La Industria de lanas en el Perú y en el departamento de Puno*, Imp. Torres Aguirre, Lima, 1929; Rory Miller, 'The Wool Trade of Southern Peru, 1850–1915', *Ibero Amerikanisches Archiv*, **8**, 1982, pp. 297–312.
3. Vicente A. Jiménez, *Apuntes Geográficos del Departamento de Puno*, Tipografía

Fournier, Puno, 1924; Eduard Dew, *Politics in the Altiplano: The Dynamics of Change in Rural Peru*, University of Texas Press, Austin, TX, 1969.

4. Wilfredo Kapsoli (ed.), *Los Movimientos campesinos en el Perú, 1879–1965*, Delva, Lima, 1977, pp. 9–80.
5. Laura L. Maltby, 'Indian Revolts in the Altiplano and the Conquest of the Land, 1895–1925', Bachelor thesis, Harvard University, 1972, p. 34.
6. Erasmo Roca, *Por la clase indígena*, Impresiones y Publicidad, Lima, 1935, p. 206; Charles Teel, 'Las raíces radicales del adventismo en el altiplano peruano', *Allpanchis*, **33**, 1989, pp. 209–48; Charles Teel, 'Missionaries, Visionaries and Revolutionaries, Logging a Passage in Search of Fernando and Ana Stahl', *Adventist Heritage*, **12**, 1988, pp. 3–14.
7. In 1940 there were 27 822 protestants in Puno, who made up 50 per cent of Peru's protestants. *Censo Nacional de Población y Ocupación de 1940*, Ministerio de Hacienda, Lima, 1944, 1, pp. 270–71. For 1915 see Jeffrey Klaiber, *La Iglesia en el Perú*, Pontificia Universidad Católica del Perú, Lima, 1988, p. 132.
8. Melchor Cutipa Coaquira, interview with the author, 1 July 1989.
9. Romero, *Monografía*, p. 382.
10. José Portugal, *José Antonio Encinas: el maestro de los maestros peruanos*, Concytec, Lima, 1986.
11. On *indigenismo* see Charles A. Hale, 'Political and Social Ideas', in Leslie Bethel (ed.), *Latin America: Economy and Society, 1870–1970*, Cambridge University Press, Cambridge, 1989, pp. 225–300.
12. Efraín Kristal, *Una Visión Urbana de los Andes: Génesis y Desarrollo del Indigenismo en el Perú, 1848–1930*, Instituto de Apoyo Agrario, Lima, 1991.
13. Marcos Cueto, 'Andean Biology in Peru: Scientific Styles in the Periphery', *Isis*, **80**, 1989, pp. 640–58.
14. David O. Wise, 'La Sierra (Lima, 1927–1930). La Voz de los Hombres del Ande', *Fénix*, **34–5**, 1989, pp. 70–105; David O. Wise, 'Vanguardismo a 3,800 metros: el caso del *Boletín Titikaka* (Puno, 1926–1930)', *Fénix*, **30–31**, 1984, pp. 257–69.
15. Luis E. Valcárcel, *Memorias*, IEP, Lima, 1981, p. 248. Rengifo, 'Esbozo biográfico de Ezequiel Urviola y Rivero', in W. Kapsoli (ed.), *Movimientos campesinos en el Perú, 1879–1965*, Delva, Lima, 1977, pp. 179–210. José Tamayo Herrera, *Historia social e indigenismo en el altiplano*, Treintaitrés, Lima, 1982.
16. According to his birth certificate he was the illegitimate child of Guillermo Núnez and Rosa Butrón. *Partida de nacimiento de Manuel María Núñez Butrón, 1 January 1899.* Testimonio de la partida de nacimiento de Manuel María Núñez Butrón, Notaría de Luis Rufasta y Banus, Barcelona, 1925, Folder Manuel Núñez Butrón, Archivo General e Histórico de la Universidad de Barcelona, Barcelona (AGHUB).
17. The biographical data are from Dan C. Hazen, 'Meanings of Literacy in the Third World: The Concepts and Consequences of the Rijchary Reform Movement in Highland Peru', *Journal of Library History*, **16**, 1981, pp. 404–15; David Frisancho Pineda, *Jatun Rijchari: Doctor Manuel Núñez Butrón, precursor de la sanidad rural en el Perú*, Los Andes, Puno, 1958; and two different collections of personal papers kept by the daughters of Núñez Butrón: Lourdes Núñez Guillén in Yanahuara, Arequipa, Papeles de Manuel Núñez Butrón, Arequipa (PMNB-A), and Rosa Jacinta Núñez in San Martín de Porres, Lima, Papeles de Manuel Núñez Butrón, Lima (PMNB-L).
18. Manuel N. Butrón, 'Necesidad del trabajo', *Esbozos, órgano de los estudiantes carolinos* (Puno), 1, 20 November 1917, 1, PMNB-L. An editorial in the journal

published by Núñez Butrón with the phrase 'it is sad to live just for the sake of it', indicates that he did not drop these ideas. Editorial, *Runa Soncco*, (*RS*), **1**, 19 May 1935, p. 1.

19. François Bourricaud, *Cambios en Puno: Estudios de Sociología andina*, Instituto Indigenista Interamericano, México, 1967. Although unsigned, the writing in the first person shows it was written by Núñez Butrón, 'Impresiones de un indio', *RS*, **3**, 24 June 1935, pp. 12–14.
20. Later, he also would also give Yanahuara as his birthplace while in Spain. *Letter from Manuel Núñez Butrón to decano de la Facultad de Medicina, 28 May 1921*, Expediente Manuel Núñez. AGHUB. Years later he received a certificate from the head of the Registro del Estado Civil in San Ramón, listing Samán as his birthplace. *Certificado de Partida de Nacimiento, March 13, 1947*, Juliaca, PMNB-L.
21. *Diario de Manuel Núnez Butrón*, no date, PMNB-L. His expenses in Spain were covered by Serafín Firpo, an Italian merchant living in Juliaca. Rosa Jacinta Núñez, interview with the author.
22. Núñez Butrón, 'Impresiones', pp. 12–14.
23. Ficha 'Núnez Butrón, Manuel', Facultad de Medicina. Registro de identidad escolar. Barcelona, 12 October 1924, AGHUB. Esteban Rodríguez Ocaña (ed.), *La Constitución de la Medicina Social como disciplina en España, 1800–1923*, Ministerio de Sanidad, Madrid, 1987; Carlos Rico-Avelló, *Historia de la Sanidad Española (1900–1925)*, Jiménez, Madrid, 1969.
24. Manuel Núñez Butrón, 'La labor cultural y sanitaria del rijchary escrito para la United Press', typewritten page, no date, PMNB-L.
25. *Censo Nacional*, 1, pp. 245–9. Alberto Ureta del Solar, 'El Saneamiento urbano en el Perú', *Boletín de la Escuela de Ingenieros del Perú*, **19**, 1946, pp. 3–76.
26. Epidemic typhus was confused with typhoid fever, and both were known as 'tabardillo'. Hermilio Valdizán and Angel Maldonado, *La Medicina Popular* (3 vols), Imp. Torres Aguirre, Lima, 1922, 2, p. 265; Juan Ayala, *Insurgencia de los Yatiris, manifestaciones culturales del hombre andino,* Concytec, Lima, 1990.
27. Valdizán and Maldonado, *La Medicina Popular*, 2, p. 24; José Marroquín, 'La medicina indígena puneña', *Anales de la Sociedad Peruana de la Historia de la Medicina*, **2**, 1940, pp. 42–57; Joseph Bastien and John Donahue, *Health in the Andes*, American Anthropological Association, Washington DC, 1981.
28. When the louse feeds on the blood of a person sick with typhus it takes the micro-organism to its stomach, where the *Rickettsia* breeds. The louse then stings a person and defecates some living micro-organisms on its skin. On scratching, the person introduces them into his blood. Charles Nicolle isolated the micro-organism in 1916. Hans Zinsser, *Rats, Lice and History, the Biography of a Bacillus*, Little Brown and Co., Boston, MA, 1934; 'Typhus, Epidemic', in Kenneth Kiple, (ed.), *Cambridge World History of Human Disease*, Cambridge University Press, Cambridge, 1993, pp. 1080–84.
29. José Marroquín, 'Estudio sanitario de un área rural en el altiplano puneño', *Salud y Bienestar Social*, **3**, 1954, p. 27; José Marroquín, *La Sanidad rural indígena en el Departamento de Puno*, Tipografía Fournier, Puno, 1945.
30. Luis Vásquez Lapeyre, 'Patología y población indígena del Perú', *Perú Indígena*, **2**, 1952, pp. 48–55; Nazario Chávez, *Cajamarca* (2 vols), Talleres Leoncio Prado, Lima, 1957, p. 212.
31. Raúl Rebagliati, 'La situación epidemiológica del Perú en 1939', *Boletín de la Dirección de Salubridad Pública*, 1940, p. 248; José Marroquín, 'Plan de acción sanitaria contra el Tifus exantemático en el Perú', *La Crónica Médica*, **66**, 1949, pp. 72–6.

32. Maxime Kuczynski Godard, *Una Inspección perliminar de las zonas del Tifus andino*, La Reforma Médica, Lima, 1940; Luis Pesce, *Indigenismo e inmigrantes en el Perú*, Imp. de la Opinión Nacional, Lima, 1906; Sebastián Lorente and Raúl Flores, *Estudios sobre Geografía Médica y Patología del Perú*, Imp. Americana, Lima, 1925.
33. Vásquez Lapeyre, 'Patología y población', p. 50.
34. Ibid., p. 49.
35. Hermilio Valdizán, *Diccionario de Medicina Peruana* (3 vols), Talleres Larco Herrera, Lima, 1923, 3, p. 204.
36. Guillermo Kuon Cabello, 'Tifus exantemático en Tarata, Tacna', *La Crónica Médica*, **66**, 1949, pp. 141–5.
37. Enrique Gamio, 'La vivienda del indio como problema nacional', *Perú Indígena*, **2**, 1952, p. 19.
38. 'Tifus exantemático; campaña permanente, organización, diciembre 2, 1931', in *Prontuario de Legislación Sanitaria del Perú* (4 vols), Imp. Americana, Lima, 1937, 2, p. 274.
39. *Variola minor*, the most common form of this disease, was known as 'mad smallpox' in the Andes and had a death rate of 1 per 100. In its other form – *Variola major* or 'black smallpox' – it had a lethality of 25–30 per cent. Valdizán and Maldonado, *Medicina Popular*, 2, p. 263. Donald Hopkins, *Princes and Peasants, Smallpox in History*, University of Chicago Press, Chicago, 1983; F. Fenner et al., *Smallpox and its Eradication*, World Health Organization, Geneva, 1988; 'Smallpox', in Kenneth Kiple (ed.), *Cambridge World History of Human Disease*, Cambridge University Press, Cambridge, 1993, pp. 1008–13.
40. Valdizán and Maldonado, *Medicina Popular*, 2, p. 263. Kaska Runa, 'La viruela en el indio altipampino', *RS*, **10**, 24 June 1948, pp. 6–8.
41. Hildebrando Castro Pozo, *Nuestra Comunidad Indígena*, El Lucero, Lima, 1924, p. 295. According to Castro Pozo, the Quechua name of smallpox was *Tayta Kapac*.
42. Juan B. Lastres, *La Salud Pública y la prevención de la viruela en el Perú*, Imp. del Ministerio de Hacienda y Comercio, Lima, 1957.
43. *Reglamento del Servicio de vacunación y revacunación antivariólicas*, Tipografía El Lucero, Lima, 1908.
44. Valdizán and Maldonado, *Medicina Popular*, 2, pp. 263–4; F. Valencia, 'Aymachura y muru', *Archivos Peruanos de Folklore*, **2**, 1953, pp. 87–90
45. 'Encuesta para conocer la epidemiología nacional, Departamento de Cajamarca', *Boletín de la Dirección de Salubridad Pública*, 1919, pp. 210–12.
46. Lorente and Flores, *Estudios*, p. 169.
47. Fenner, et al., *Smallpox*, pp. 333, 601. An important factor was that the price of the vaccine fell. Julio Portugal, 'La sanidad en el Perú', *Boletín de la Dirección de Salubridad Pública*, 1947; Carlos Bouroncle Díaz, 'Vacunación contra la viruela en el Perú en los últimos veinte años', Bachelor thesis, Universidad Nacional Mayor de San Marcos, 1970, p. 33.
48. José Marroquín, 'El problema sanitario Indígena en Puno', *Medicina Social*, **2**, 1944, p. 6.
49. Abel Olaechea, 'Breve estudio de la situación higiénica y asistencia del Perú en el período comprendido desde fines del siglo XVII y la época presente', *Revista Médica Peruana*, **5**, 1933, p. 630.
50. 'Por qué no salen los médicos a provincias', *La Acción Médica*, **6**, 4 February 1928, p. 12.
51. In some provinces the physicians resigned their appointment when forced to

move to the countryside. *Efraín Trelles, Jefe de la V Concentración Sanitaria Regional a Prefecto del Cuzco, 14 July and 22 August 1938*, Serie Prefectura Cuzco, Subserie Comunicaciones, Leg. 13, Year 1938, Archivo Departamental del Cuzco, Cuzco (ADCu).

52. Manuel Núñez Butrón, '¿Qué es el Rijcharismo?', *Medicina Social*, **2**, 1944, pp. 9–10.
53. This happened even though state physicians were forbidden to sell medicines in 1941. *Prontuario de Legislación Sanitoria del Perú*, (4 vols), Imp. Americana, Lima, 1937, 4, pp. 544–6.
54. 'La Gran Cruzada Sanitaria', *Medicina Social*, **9**, 1952, pp. 10–13.
55. Luis E. Valcárcel, *Tempestad en los Andes*, Minerva, Lima, 1927.
56. 'El nombramiento *Rijchary*, 1937', and Manuel Núñez Butrón, 'La sanidad rural en el departamento de Puno', *RS*, **7**, 24 June 1937, pp. 29 and 12.
57. Un *rijchary*, 'Labor *rijchary*', *RS*, **10**, 24 June 1948, p. 10.
58. Mariano Velásquez García, interview, 27 June 1989.
59. Rebagliati, 'La situación', pp. 261–2.
60. *Prontuario*, 2, pp. 31–2.
61. 'Labor de los sanitarios *rijcharys* de la brigada', *RS*, **7**, 24 June 1937, p. 32.
62. Joseph Bastien, *Healers of the Andes: Kallawaya Herbalists and the Medical Plants*, University of Utah Press, Salt Lake City, UT, 1987.
63. 'La Fiesta del Indio en la capital de nuestra provincia', *RS*, **4**, 28 July 1935, pp. 14–15.
64. An index of the pharmaceutical growth was the establishment, in 1943, of the Inspección General de Farmacia in the Ministry of Health.
65. A. Mollepasa, 'Lo que quiere decir Runa Soncco', *RS*, **6**, 30 January 1937, p. 1. The journal bore the subtitle of 'the eventual journal of *Rijchary* rural health', and the 'director responsible' was Núñez Butrón. A complete collection of this journal is in the National Library of Lima. A list of the issues and publishing dates of the journal according to the journal itself, is as follows:

Volume or year	Issue	Date
1	1	April 1935
1	2	19 May 1935
1	3	24 June 1935
1	4	28 July 1935
1	5	30 September 1935
3	6	30 January 1937
3	7	24 June 1937
11	8	September 1945
12	9	April 1946
14	10	24 June 1948

66. 'Editorial', *RS*, **1**, April 1935, p. 1.
67. Ministerio de Hacienda e Commercio, *Estado de la Instrucción en el Perú según el censo nacional de 1940*, Imp. Torres Aguirre, Lima, 1942, p. 47.
68. 'Viruela', *RS*, **4**, 28 July 1935, pp. 10–11; Carlos Amauta, 'El tifus exantemático', *RS*, **8**, September 1945, p. 32.
69. Inty Sonhon, 'En el mundo de los piojos', *RS*, **8**, September 1945, p. 6.
70. Kaska Runa, 'La viruela', p. 8. According to another article, the brigade reformed the methods of traditional medicine until 'they finally had a scientific basis'. 'Un *rijchary*', *RS*, **10**, 24 June 1948, p. 11.
71. 'Viruela', *RS*, **1**, April 1935, p. 11.
72. *Censo nacional*, p. 147.

73. 'Biblioteca ambulante *rijchary*', *RS*, **3**, 30 January 1937, p. 9; 'Reunión, 12 July, 1953', Cuaderno de Actas *Rijchary*, PMNB-A; 'Orientaciones pedagógicas, la enseñanza de la aritmética en la escuela indígena', *RS*, **4**, 28 July 1935, p. 13.
74. 'Himno Nacional del Perú', *RS*, **7**, 24 June 1937, p. 1.
75. A. Mollepasa, 'Sobre el aseo', *RS*, **7**, 24 June 1937, p. 9.
76. 'El nombramiento *rijchary*', p. 29.
77. *RS*, **7**, 24 June 1937, p. 14.
78. 'Palabras amigas', *RS*, **5**, 30 September 1935, p. 13.
79. Capitalized in the original, 'Runa Soncco', *RS*, **6**, 30 January 1937, p. 25.
80. Howard Handelman, *Struggle in the Andes: Peasant Political Mobilization in Peru*, University of Texas Press, Austin, TX, 1975, p. 31.
81. *Gamonales* was a name used in the Andes for those landowners or *hacendados* who ran their rural estates in brutal and primitive fashion. *Cholos* was used for Indians who tried to whiten their culture.
82. *RS*, **7**, 24 June 1937, p. 22; and the article signed by Y.B.O., 'Lápiz Rojo', in the same issue, p. 18.
83. Gabriel Delgado Bedoya, 'Doctrina y acción *rijchary* de Manuel Núñez Butrón', *Medicina Social*, **10**, 1953, p. 9.
84. *Presidente de la República to Director de Salubridad, 19 November 1937*; *Efraín Trelles to Manuel Núnez Butrón, 29 November 1937*; *Letter of the Sección Administrativa de la Dirección de Salubridad to Manuel Núñez Butrón, 7 May 1938*, PMNB-L.
85. According to the 'Relación nominal de los señores médicos-cirujanos conforme al censo practicado de 1940', *Boletín de la Directión de Salubridad Publica*, 1940, p. 184, Núñez Butrón lived in Juliaca in 1940.
86. The quotes figure as mottoes in *RS*, **9**, April 1946, p. 34; 'Vuelve *Runa Soncco*', *RS*, **8**, September 1945, p. 1.
87. The article figured as an interview with Andrés Lampa Mamani. 'Como habla el indio de hoy', *RS*, **10**, 24 June 1948, p. 47.
88. The leaflet is '*Carta abierta. Manuel Núñez Butrón, Juliaca, 1 June, 1946*', PMNB-A.
89. Another leaflet is 'Una de nuestras representaciones que merece apoyo', and another said he had not 'been concerned with obtaining a personal benefit from the misery of his fellow beings'; it was titled 'Dr. Manuel Núñez Butrón' and was signed by the 'Comité de la Unión San Román', PNMB-L.
90. *RS*, **10**, 24 June 1948, p. 1.
91. José Tamayo Herrera, *Historia del Indigenismo Cuzqueño, siglos XVI–XX*, INC, Lima, 1980, p. 255; Tamayo Herrera, *Historia social e indigenismo*.
92. *Letter of Manuel Núñez Butrón to Carlos Alberto Butrón, Juliaca, 1 December 1952*, PMNB-A.
93. However, Núñez Butrón declared that if he was given the choice between a mansion in Paris and a house in Juliaca, he would choose the latter. Told by Juan Molina in 'Reunión, julio 12, 1953', Cuadernos de Actas, PMNB-A.
94. The data in 'Manuel Núñez Butrón contra Lidia Cabrera sobre divorcio absoluto, 31 May, 1935', *Actuario Luis Rosado*, Expedientes Judiciales 1935, Leg. 1261, Archivo Departamental de Puno, Puno (ADPu).
95. 'Copia simple del testamento otorgado por el Dr. Manuel Núñez Butrón a favor de sus hijos', Varios actuarios. Expedientes judiciales 1940–50, Leg. 224–36, ADPu.
96. Rosa Jacinta Núnez, interview.
97. 'Labor sanitaria durante el presente mes', *RS*, **4**, 28 July 1935, p. 3. Similar measures were taken in other provinces. In Cuzco, certificates of vaccination

were requested to buy train tickets. *Alfredo Arteta a Prefecto, 31 October 1948*, Serie Prefectura Cuzco, Subserie Comunicaciones, Leg. 19, Year 1948, ADCu.

98. The journal published an interview with Núñez Butrón in 'La Gran Cruzada', pp. 10–13.

CHAPTER FOUR

The Recurring Burden of Malaria

Some diseases are accepted as part of everyday life because of their scope and frequency. In Peru, malaria is certainly one of these. The terms *chujcho* (Quechua), paludism, *calenturas*, *tembladera*, *tercianas*, and *quartana*, were associated to symptoms of the disease such as the intermittent combination of shivers, fever and perspiration which usually do not kill but weaken patients, leaving them unable to work and susceptible to the development of other diseases. Malaria, a disease caused by the *Plasmodium* parasite which is transmitted by the *Anopheles* mosquito, abounds in Peru. Of the three forms in which the *Plasmodium* parasite is found in this country, *vivax*, *malarie* and *falciparum*, the first is the most frequent and goes under the name of *terciana* or benign malaria, while the latter is the only one which causes a rapid death.[1]

Two characteristics of the history of malaria in Peru are, first, that it reinforced cultural and geographical variants and, second, that the campaigns against the disease had an impact on the meaning of public health in Peru.

The ecological and social bases

In Peru, malaria has traditionally been considered a typical disease of the coast and the Amazon forest. Although the division into coast, highlands and Amazon forest is criticized by some geographers, this classification was long used to divide Peru according to its altitude above sea level and its relation to the Andean cordillera.[2] For instance, the coast is regarded as going from 0 to 1500 metres above sea level, and the Amazon forest begins and climbs down the eastern slopes of the Andes at 2000 metres above sea level.[3] The separation of these three areas is useful to understand the ecological basis of malaria. There are some geographical and environmental characteristics – like altitude, rainfall periodicity and volume, river beds – which are quite definitely prone to malaria but which differ on the coast and in the Amazon basin, and are missing in the highlands.[4]

Except at its northernmost tip, the coast is criss-crossed by small valleys separated by desert areas where rains are unusual. The rivers forming these valleys flow down from the surrounding Andes at a steep gradient. In the rainy season (January to March) they swell, their bed becomes erratic and drags sand, earth and stones that form swamps and other water deposits. The larvae of

Anopheles grow in stagnant waters, which increase towards the end of the rainy season.

Other environmental factors which favour the growth of mosquitoes on the coast are its moderate temperature, usually over 16°C, and a high humidity of about 70 per cent, which helps *Anopheles* develop in almost every season, particularly in late summer when the rainy season in the highlands is over. A characteristic of this mosquito is that it is not usually found in Peru over 1500 metres above sea level.[5] Those years with unusually heavy rains on the coast (such as 1925 and 1926) create better conditions for transmission of the disease due to the increase in the number of reservoirs, but spectacular outbreaks of malaria rarely take place.

The most common *Anopheles* in the coastal and highland valleys is the *A. pseudopunctipennis*, whose females suck people's blood to get proteins and help their eggs mature; they lay their eggs in shallow reservoirs with algae on the banks on which the sun shines. The breeding grounds in the lower part of the valleys disappear in the dry season. The mosquitoes then remain in ponds, water puddles and backwaters of stony rivers located at higher altitudes until the rains form new breeding grounds in the lower part of the valleys.[6] In brief, on the coast the environmental factors favourable for malaria are a moderate temperature, high humidity, a low altitude and the seasonality of the rains in the highlands.[7]

Neither the *Anopheles* nor the natural transmission of malaria exist in most of the highlands due to the cold climate, the dry environment, the altitude and the ruggedness of the land which prevents water from stagnating. However, there are imported cases of malaria brought from the coast, the Amazon forest or the highland valleys. The ecological foundations of malaria are different in the Amazon, where rivers are bigger and rains more persistent, from those on the coast. The season with least malaria is that with the highest rainfall (from June to August) because the intensity of the rains impedes the preservation of the larvae breeding grounds. The river flow diminishes in the dry season and swamps and ponds where the larvae live are formed.[8] The rains are frequent and life is hard for the *Anopheles* in low altitude areas above sea level. The variety of mosquitoes is greater in the Amazon basin than on the coast, and the major vectors are *A. darlingi, rangeli* and *oswaldoi*. Finally, malaria worsens in the Amazon basin due to intestinal infections like hookworm disease, the lack of medical services, crops that require flooding, like rice and *gramalote* (a low-quality grass for cattle), the destruction of the forest, the poor condition of canals, reservoirs and irrigation canals, excavations made while building houses, paths, roads and irrigation works, and some customs pertaining to the storage of water that favour the growth of *Anopheles*, such as having wells near dwellings.[9]

A human factor related to malaria in Peru was the migration between different geographical regions. Malaria was unforgiving for migrants from the highlands who reached the coast and the Amazon. This was because malaria bestows a limited immunity where it is endemic in nature, as on the coast and the Amazon forest, where many endure it from childhood. Individuals acquire a relative protection from later infections if they survive the disease at an age when it is not particularly severe.[10] Immunity can also be attained after several infections, which leave behind a wake of poor health and anaemia. In contrast, the people from the highlands who migrated to the coastlands or to the Amazon forest for trade or seasonal agricultural work had no previous experience with *Plasmodium*. According to Peruvian physicians, malaria was a childhood disease among the natives of the Amazon forest 'which dies out slowly during growth', while foreigners behaved 'like children' before malaria.[11] This perception is confirmed with data from 1956, which indicate that malaria particularly attacked young men of working age, thus suggesting that the disease was related to migration.[12]

Migration from the highlands to the coast and the Amazon forest increased in the early twentieth century with the expansion of rural estates and firms dedicated to the commercialization of sugar, rice, wood, fruits and rubber, and the rise in the number of rural workers. The coastlands always had scant labour, and attempts were made to solve this through several labour systems (like the import of Chinese labourers in the early nineteenth century).[13] In the early twentieth century, the labour needs of the coastal *haciendas* were covered by *enganche* Indians. Highland labourers always worked during the planting season and the harvest, which coincided with the highest incidence of *Anopheles*.[14] There was also a seasonal migration of people from the highlands in relation to trade, fairs, religious festivals and road building. Besides their lack of experience with *Plasmodium*, highlanders who caught malaria had to contend with difficult access to traditional or western medicine, the absence of a family on whom they could rely, the exploitation they were subject to and their terrible living conditions.[15] Highlanders were also taken to the *haciendas* in the tropical forest because it was believed that natives did not work in a disciplined way. There was a higher risk for foreigners and some immunity for natives, just like on the coast.

These factors all helped develop an idea among early twentieth-century Peruvian physicians, geographers and writers that a connection existed between malaria and the Indians who worked in the coastal and Amazon rural estates.[16] Many of them believed that the people who caught malaria were from the highlands. This was interpreted as a sign of racial impairment, or as the reason behind the underdevelopment of agriculture and the poverty of the Indians.[17] Some examples of this current of thought are: Francisco Graña, the first Professor of Hygiene at the University of San Marcos, who considered in 1916 that malaria was a 'barrier that limits the immigration of Indians to the coast'. In the 1920s, health officials likewise stated that the rural labourers from the highland working on the coast 'almost invariably' caught malaria.[18]

The connection between geographical locations and some diseases was not new, but with malaria it gained a new lease among Peruvian physicians. The researcher Pedro Weiss restated the connection between ecological sites, migratory currents and some endemic diseases. His studies stressed the significance disease-gendered environmental barriers had in dividing the geographical regions of Peru. As for malaria, he repeated what must have then been a commonplace: 'The paludic coast has for centuries been a cemetery for highlanders.'[19]

The connection between migrant labour and malaria extended beyond Lima. For example, in 1918 the physician in the coastal locality of Huacho explained that malaria particularly attacked 'the rural workers from the *haciendas* ... who come from the highlands and live in terrible conditions of hygiene'.[20] The state physician of Lambayeque, an essentially rice-producing area, likewise believed in 1915 that coast dwellers were 'immune to paludism'.[21] Some coastal physicians considered there was a natural proclivity to the disease in the Indians, which was of more importance than the social and ecological factors. According to a physician in Ica, malaria came to the valley with the summer and so did:

> [a] great number of labourers from the highlands ... Their poor type of food, the inborn idiosyncrasy of the highlanders, and their misleading coca chewing are factors that place them in ideal conditions to get paludism. After two or three weeks this man, who can still resist his severe attacks of malaria, goes to the hospital exhausted and pauperized with a host of complications, where tuberculosis in particular predominates.[22]

Physicians in the highlands likewise perceived the vulnerability of the Indians. In reply to a poll distributed by the health authorities, the state physician of Yungay, which is 2585 metres above sea level, reported in 1917 that malaria was imported from the coast 'especially by the Indians returning from work in the *haciendas*'.[23] The state physician of Cajamarca, from where the *enganche* labourers for the rice crops of Lambayeque came, likewise denounced in 1915 that malaria, which had previously been an occasional disease, was 'now an illness that sends a great number of patients to the men's hospital', and that when these workers could no longer stay on the coast they returned to the highlands 'weakened, terribly anaemic due to paludism, to be interned in the hospital of this city'.[24]

The peculiarities malaria had in Peru were also perceived by the people themselves. When writing about a coastal city, one writer pointed out that the vectors of malaria and typhus distinguished the coast from the highlands: 'Just like Indians are louse meat in our highlands, so the mestizos are *zancudo* [a name for the mosquito] meat in Chiclayo and in almost all of the coast.'[25] For the people on the coast, living side by side with a great number of mosquitoes was taken as a matter of fact, and a way to identify foreigners was when one complained of the insects or had a high fever. Some forms of medication show an adaptation to the disease. For instance, during the malaria epidemics of Loreto in the early twentieth century, people preferred to have their children get the disease to prevent later and stronger infections.[26] Other manifestations of the popular perceptions of the disease are the name given to malaria ('valley disease') and the fact that it was not easy getting labourers to work in the tropical forest because 'convinced they are going to their death, each day they are more reluctant to migrate to the lowland forest'.[27] The lyrics to a song from the highland town of Chota (Cajamarca), in the northern Andes, show that the highland labourers were aware of the dangers present in their migratory displacements:

> Chotatino peasant
> You help yourself on the coast
> there you sweat without feeling it
> and return to your hut
> to die sick with tuberculosis.[28]

The Indians of Paucartambo and Apurímac believed malaria was a disease of muleteers, the merchants who carried goods from one valley to the next. In Paucartambo there was a dance of the *palúdicos* (those sick with malaria) where muleteers danced with yellow masks as a metaphor of the paleness that comes with anaemia.[29] In Apurímac it was believed that one caught the disease after seeing a beautiful mestiza with a red petticoat, a straw hat and a green blouse sitting close to the river. A physician deconstructed this vision connecting 'the red with the fever, green with the Amazon forest, and the colour of straw with malarial paleness'.[30]

Malaria did not just reveal perceptions, identities and stigmas. It also gave rise to public debates and policies on agricultural development, Amazon colonization, and social service.

The first campaigns

The campaigns waged by the Peruvian government against malaria in the twentieth century fall into two phases. The first began at the turn of the century and lasted until the 1940s. The second phase goes from the 1940s to the failure of eradication in the 1970s. Larvae control and treating the sick were the goals of the first period. Larvae were controlled through expensive hydraulic works such as the drainage of water tanks, or spraying them with substances like Paris green or petrol, which prevented the larvae from breathing on the surface. The fumigation and protection of dwellings with mosquito netting and wire frames were complementary measures.

For the sick, medication consisted in administering quinine through drugs. Peru imported quinine from at least 1928 even though the plant was native to the Andes.[31] However, its amount and quality was not always adequate, medication was expensive and it required rest, for which there was not always time. Quinine was accepted by the coastal people as a palliative for the fever. According to a physician, 'There are individuals who on finding they have contracted malaria ... take ... quinine and then go back to their work'.[32] The sporadic medications nonetheless helped make the disease chronic.

The first step taken by the State to control malaria came with the 1916 Law 2364, known as Prophylaxis against Malaria, which was due to an outbreak in Chanchamayo. According to the law, the landowners (*hacendados*) should protect their workers, give them free quinine, and destroy the larvae. The law exempted quinine and wire frames from all taxes, and laid down the minimum distance allowed between habitations and rice and sugar cane fields.[33] Some landowners complied, particularly on the north and central coast, with the part on providing a medical service, and also supplied quinine and cleaned irrigation canals. Less common was having swamps drained because these were considered 'irrigation tanks', or having the workers' lodges rebuilt. After an outbreak in Chanchamayo, one of the areas colonized in the Amazon forest, the landowners formed a Philanthropical Society which from 1908 to 1918 managed a hospital for patients with malaria.[34] The government later supported the hospital, but charging the landowners for the treatment of their employees proved difficult. In general, the enforcement of the law was erratic, and gave rise to a situation where the State and the landowners wanted to attract migrants but were unable to defray the costs involved in sanitation.

The anti-malarial bills stirred a debate that disclosed the conflicting interests involved in the control of the disease. For instance, a common debate hinged on what should be the distance between rice fields and settlements. The physicians tried to have the landowners shoulder all responsibility and backed the 2 kilometres established in the bill. The rice producers were a more cohesive group than the landowners in the highlands but had less influence than the sugar planters; their influence sprung from the fact that rice was an essential staple in the Peruvian diet – its cultivation had been protected by tariffs since the turn of the twentieth century, and the area under cultivation had grown since then. The controversy caused a debate between physicians and rice producers. In 1932, the National Medical Academy released a statement prepared by Carlos Enrique Paz Soldán, warning of the malarial threat posed by rice. The landowners replied with a statement prepared by the Rice Conference held that same year, declaring there had never been a mono-causal connection between rice and malaria, and criticized the compulsory execution of sanitation works.[35]

The dispute reached the halls of a private club, where the agricultural engineer and landowner Gerardo Klinge and the physician Paz Soldán continued the debate. Klinge insisted that a study of the mosquitoes which transmitted malaria in Peru was needed, and pointed out the malarial responsibility of sugar cane, which required periodic irrigation, and cotton, which needed puddles in the irrigation ditches. For Klinge there was no direct relationship with the crop; each valley instead had malarial and non-malarial areas which the population was aware of, and an anti-malarial bill was utopian because there was no way in which all mosquitoes could be destroyed. Finally, he argued that rice cultivation could not be eradicated because that would cause unemployment and hunger. His conclusion was definitive: 'If rice is an evil, then it must be admitted that it is a necessary evil.'[36]

These debates did not take place in other areas, nor could the law be enforced due to the weakness of the medical profession and the State. In 1940, for example, the state physician visited the malarial areas of Ayacucho (Huanta, La Mar and Cangallo) and concluded he could not ask the landowners to 'give medical assistance … because of the lack of professionals in this region'.[37] In that same year the people of Acón, in Huanta, denounced that the representative of the Anti-Malarial Service had not visited them. The accused replied he did not have transport, and that the number of patients was too high.[38]

Other problems the physicians had to contend with were resistance and the refusal to admit one was sick. For many mothers, the malarial fever of their children was no more than a 'scare'. There was a widespread belief that malaria was caught by being too long in the water or eating unripe fruits, and that the best treatment for it was to take infusions of bitter herbs to 'extract the cold' or 'scare' the patients. It was also believed that demons or sprites who made the travellers sick lived in ponds, ravines and in some parts of the rivers. For protection there were some objects and rituals that had to be complied with when passing through those places. Avoiding these areas at the time mosquitoes abounded was also recommended. Due to incidents of incomplete medication with quinine and to the fact that high doses had toxic effects, physicians in the tropical forest had to prescribe the drug under another name 'so it cannot be identified'.[39] The workers in coastal rural estates had a strong reason to deny having malaria: they were afraid of losing their jobs.[40]

By 1939, the Ministry of Health estimated that the annual number of people sick with malaria was 300 000. It likewise deplored the fact that control of the disease was 'scant, almost non-existent', and that in some areas malaria was 'something … no one protests about nor deplores; it is accepted as a fact of life'.[41] The limitations of the traditional resources were described in the following terms: 'paludism will not vanish as long as waters are not channelled … as long as swamp lands are not drained, tasks which physicians do not know how to do'.[42] The exposed condition of the people and the weakness of institutions in the face of malaria are shown by a horrendous malaria outbreak that ravaged a valley in Cuzco in 1932.

An epidemic in La Convención

When the road reached Quillabamba in late 1932, its people could not refrain from celebrating it with a dance in the manor house of the *hacienda* Macamango. Some surely did so under the impression that it was the last time they would celebrate, not because there would be nothing left to celebrate in future, but because that very day a dreadful malaria epidemic had also arrived. In a metaphor for the strange coincidence of modernity and disease which sometimes happens, those who were celebrating the arrival of the road danced in the same building whose cellar housed the first victims of the epidemic.[43] Thus began the worst malaria outbreak in twentieth-century Peru.

Quillabamba, the provincial capital of La Convención, one of the largest and least populated provinces of Peru with an area of 105 122 square kilometres, was founded in the late nineteenth century and gained the status of town only in 1918. The province, located in the department of Cuzco, had the same name as the valley formed by the great Urubamba River. The area had an abrupt prosperity in the early twentieth century due to its integration in the markets of Cuzco, Puno and Bolivia supplying coca, sugar and food. This was part of the process of consolidation of a southern wool network in which cities like Arequipa, Puno and Cuzco each had a complementary role. While credit managed by wholesale firms abounded in the first city, the second concentrated its efforts in the production of wool, and the agricultural produce of the upper Urubamba valley was sold in the third, an area which witnessed a striking increase in its number of rural estates thanks to the laws passed in 1898 and 1909 favouring the colonization of lowland tropical forest lands.[44] The greatest revenue in the region accrued from coca, sugar and cane liquor. By the time of the epidemic, land under coca claimed 42.7 per cent of the 6700 hectares cultivated in the valley of La Convención, which provisioned Cuzco and other Andean departments. Food supplies (cassava, maize, bananas, and other fruits), sugar cane, cacao and coffee respectively took up 29.8 per cent, 11.9 per cent, 10.4 per cent and 5.9 per cent of the hectares under cultivation.[45] These products were grown in *haciendas* with little capital or technology, whose owners lived in relative luxury in the city of Cuzco.

The harsh living conditions in lands which were not just uncultivated but were also located in narrow ravines, the resistance shown by the natives of the forest (the Machiguengas) to becoming peasants and the distance between cultivated lands and any settlement, all impeded the development of a free labour market or recourse to the *enganche* system. The landowners in La Convención found a solution to the lack of labour in peasants who were also settlers, supervised by foremen living in the valley. In this system, the owners leased the *haciendas* to tenants in return for a series of obligations which included working in the lands and house of the owner. The tenants usually signed a nine-year contract. According to this agreement, the lease was not paid the first year as it was invested in preparing the land. As the quality and the output of the land rose, so did the amount the owner received as lease.[46] The tenants in turn subleased plots of land to relatives in return for work and produce. The tenants usually fulfilled their obligations with the landowner through their relatives. These tasks comprised sending servants to the home of their employer, and providing journeymen who worked some days each month in the lands of the landowner. The contracts stipulated not just the work of men but also of women, which was valuable during the harvest. The agricultural peons were the lowest rung in this system of personal dependence, had no land and worked for short periods of time in the *hacienda* or on the lands of the tenants or of a relative. Payments made to the peons were in cash, liquor and food. Finally, there was a floating population of muleteers and merchants in the region who went to and from the city of Cuzco.

Living conditions both in the *haciendas* and on the land worked by peasants were extremely poor. The living quarters prepared to house the *hacienda* workers temporarily were 'dark, filthy rooms [and] were never disinfected'.[47] Peasants had to defray all improvements made in their lands and homes without any reimbursement from the owner. The destitution of peasant life appears in a contemporary source:

> Their dwelling consists of huts made of straw and sticks, a kind of cage with bars just a few centimetres one from the other. In them live people of all sexes and ages in great promiscuity, together with their animals ... The same room serves as kitchen ... They usually sleep on some kind of makeshift bedsteads made of straw ... others just lie on the floor ...[48]

According to one writer, the settlement system promoted by the *haciendas* was an inefficient solution to the need for commercial expansion in the tropical forest, particularly because of the lack of a social infrastructure to support colonization.[49] The destitution of rural workers was not just due to a colonization system bereft of sanitation. Besides this, the presence of the State was barely felt in La Convención. Until the late 1920s, this was a frontier area of the department of Cuzco where the fragility of its municipal institutions and its small police force were in stark contrast to the smugglers, bandits and fugitives who hid in the valley. Municipal institutions were further debilitated by their erratic revenues, poor management and the frequent turnover of authorities. The municipal council barely met and blamed their poor conditions on the roads and the little incentive there was to hold a municipal post.[50]

In the midst of this lack of authority, one institution had legitimacy and ascendancy over the people: the Dominican Order. The Dominican missionaries arrived in 1903 with the rubber boom in the tropical forest. They were joined in the 1920s by the nuns of the order, who opened a school for girls in Quillabamba. The ascendancy attained by the Dominicans was due to their devotion and persistence, their ascetic way of life and the attention they paid to the people's overall problems. According to Sabas Sarasola, the Spanish parish priest of Quillabamba, when evangelizing, people had to be turned into human beings before making them Christians.[51] However, neither the Dominicans nor the landowners were prepared for malaria. The oldest inhabitants recalled epidemics in 1898 and 1902, but none as 'resistant' as that of 1932.[52]

The outbreak began in one of the most distant parts of the area under colonization. The first cases appeared in August 1932 in Siriato, within the land of the Machiguenga tribes and close to the Dominican missions of Coribeni and then moved up river until it reached more densely populated towns. Alarmed by the rapid spread of the disease, the bishop, the mayor and other authorities of Quillabamba met and requested help to face an 'unknown epidemic which is causing a great many deaths'.[53] The news in the Cuzco daily papers was appalling:

> People newly arrived from the villages of Sahuayaco, Chacanares, Chaco, Roroncoe and Sajiruyo report ... the sick in each village are several score; that fearing contagion, the relatives of the sick emigrate in all directions in an endless exodus, leaving their relatives to their fate. The huts of these forlorn people are abandoned and the bodies left unburied, to be eaten by ravens.[54]

In the ensuing months the news of roads that could not be used due to the stench of abandoned corpses spread like wildfire. The distance between dwellings, the lack of roads and poverty, all made a physician remark that the inhabitants were 'not even ready to die'.[55] Samuel Geller, the state physician of La Convención, ascertained that Echerate, some 35 kilometres from Quillabamba, was the district most affected by the epidemic.[56] He also established that the epidemic hit the children hard but adults too, which showed the disease was new for the people.

At first it was believed that the epidemic could be yellow fever, for the sick died in 24 hours with vomiting, a high fever, headaches and a pale countenance.[57] (The most common form of malaria is characterized by an intermittent fever which does not kill immediately.) Although the provincial state physician believed it was malaria, only entomological and haematological samples could ascertain the identity of the disease. Luis Ugarte, the state physician of the department of Cuzco, did not find the vector for yellow fever, and Johannes Willie, a member of a scientific committee sent from Lima found the *Anopheles pseudopunctipennis*, which he considered was the agent transmitting malaria. Ugarte declared having found in blood tests the '*Plasmodium falciparum*, the agent of malignant malaria ... and also ... benign paludism or the tertian form'.[58] The National Medical Academy agreed with Ugarte and declared the roots of the epidemic probably lay in the 'chronic' malaria of the jungle tribes. Although the presence of *Plasmodium falciparum* was never confirmed, epidemiological and clinical data indicate the epidemic was caused by this parasite.[59]

The absence of a more precise identification of the disease was also due to how critical the situation was. For many it was no more than an ailment that caused 'severe headaches, high fevers and ... left people as weak and run-down as if they had been sick for a whole month, and few were able to avoid relapse'.[60] In 1944 a university student visited Quello-Mayo, close to the *hacienda* Huadquiña, and described a scene that probably was not different from the situation in 1932:

> On entering this dwelling we are seized with horror and fear before death ... two or three men appear before us, extended on their sick bed with only a poncho as bed, men who wail and are shivering to the point where their teeth chatter ... They are so weakened ... they have no strength left ... even to see who has just entered [their home] ... pale countenaces, yellow, weak ... in a word, they look like human spectres. If we ask them what they have, they weakly reply: 'paludism is shaking me'.[61]

The epidemic moved rapidly up river and went from low-altitude areas to the Andean ranges. According to the state physician from Calca, there was an inverse relation between the epidemic and altitude. The number of cases increased as one went down into the jungle, and was less in the highest rural estates of the valley. Interestingly, the epidemic was preceded by heavy rains which multiplied the breeding grounds of the mosquitoes.[62]

The colonization of the Amazon forest itself played a part in the origins of the epidemic. It was usual for peasants to burn the forest so as to make it cultivatable, a procedure known as slash and burn.[63] Deforestation is one of the causes of malaria because it allows the rain to make water reservoirs. Road-building, which increased just before the epidemic, likewise left behind swamps and puddles that became breeding grounds. The high death rate and rapid spread of the epidemic can be explained by flight from infected areas, the passage of merchants and the mobility of rural labourers.

This mobility was decisive for the spread of malaria, as is borne out by the fact that the first cases were of people who entered the tropical forests and then returned to their settlements, and that workers travelled from their homes in the upper reaches of the valley to the lands of the landowners, usually located at a lower altitude where mosquitoes abounded. Malaria was also spread by the muleteers who frequently travelled all through the valley peddling their goods and leading highland labourers who were not acquainted with the disease. The relatives, tenants and agricultural peons were usually Indians from the highlands of Cuzco, Apurímac, Puno, Arequipa and Ayacucho, where malaria was unknown. According to one Dominican friar, the epidemic was particularly virulent with 'the *puñarunas*, i.e. Indians from the highlands who had come to these lands to earn their living'.[64] The low incidence of malaria among the natives of the Amazon forest was because the adult members of the tribes had some immunity. Physicians believed the natives would not spread the disease because of their immunity, and because they had scant contact with the outside world. On the other hand, migration and colonization caused health problems for the natives of the tropical forest. These fell victim to diseases unknown to them, like smallpox and influenza, which were caught by natives who travelled to the highlands in search of salt and other goods.[65]

The depopulation brought about by malaria was due to the lack of work, food and a generalized famine. They who survived malaria usually fell prey to tuberculosis, smallpox and other no less deadly diseases. Conditions in the valley were calamitous towards the end of the epidemic. According to the landowners: 'there are not enough workers, the lands are not cultivated ... plots of land become forests where wild animals live, and domestic animals go wild'.[66] The epidemic put the Dominican friars, the municipalities, the landowners and the State to the test.

One sign of the inability of the authorities to organize a campaign was the state of the Quillabamba town council, which was vacant in November 1933 due to the resignation of eight aldermen. There likewise were no councilmen in Lares from July to December 1933, only the mayor was left.[67] These vacancies were probably due to the flight of the authorities themselves. The subprefect of La Convención established a mandatory obligation to act *ad honorem* as lieutenant-governor by turns. Some protested the imposition, and the fact that the post entailed collecting and isolating the sick.[68] On the other hand, the mayor of Lares decided to drain swamps and ponds through compulsory public works. Since it was not easy getting the support of the landowners, the mayor fined all who failed to comply with his decree. However, on finding he could not collect the fine the mayor transferred the responsibility for controlling the epidemic to other provincial and departmental authorities.[69]

The weakness of the regional authorities, the half-hearted measures taken by the State, and the scant intervention of the landowners increased the importance of the Dominican friars. The nuns of the order improvised a hospital in a school which looked after 2770 patients between November 1932 and December 1934.[70] In that period, the hospital's expenditures were defrayed by the Dominicans, some landowners and a group of ladies from the Anti-Malarial League of Cuzco. The number of patients was so high that patients were taken only when they had a fever and then returned home with some indications on how to avoid relapsing.

Dejection and helplessness heightened the religiosity of the people, a feeling the Dominicans fostered. The religious fervor was visible in the great Mass held when the hospital of Quillabamba opened. Displaying his ability as an orator in the ceremony, Father Sarasola begged 'for heavenly mercy' and 'exhorted the sick to ... penitence'.[71] A great painting was placed at the entrance, over the Eucharist, titled *Merciful Love*. In early 1933 the triduum was held in Quillabamba, a three-day period of penance that reached its climax in an imposing procession where the faithful walked with 'crosses, small crosses, big crosses, chanting sad dirges in Quechua and Spanish whose lyrics pain the heart with their verses of repentance and forgiveness'.[72] The most dramatic moment came when the procession reached the hospital and a mother who was breast-feeding her baby fell dead with malaria. Religiosity spread all over Cuzco, where a procession was held headed by the authorities and the image of the Lord of Earthquakes.[73] According to the sermons preached by the Dominicans, the root of the epidemic lay in the sins of the people and healing required repentance. These sermons must have been favourably received by the people.

Religion was also important because there was no official response. Although news of the epidemic had reached Lima in November 1932, it was only in late December – partly because no one was then in charge of the Bureau of Public Health – that the first measures were taken and La Convención and Lares were declared malarial.[74] The belated response of the government was due to the political crisis Peru was going through at the time under the administration of Commander Luis Sánchez Cerro, who took office in December 1931. The instability of the administration worsened with the charges of electoral fraud, the Aprista uprising in northern Peru, the sailors' mutiny in Callao, an aborted attempt against the life of the President, the closing of the University of San Marcos, an aborted *coup d'état*, a frontier incident with Colombia that almost ended in open war and, finally, the murder of Sánchez Cerro in April 1933.

Political instability therefore explains why the administration wanted to downplay the epidemic. According to Alberto Giesecke, president of Cuzco University, Sánchez Cerro had stated that the epidemic was a matter of 'no importance' and ordered the newspapers to refrain from touching the subject.[75] However, this could not conceal how serious the situation was. In mid-1933, Sarasola complained of the indifference shown in the face of such a great death toll, and revealed that the shipments of quinine were not even enough for 20 per cent of the sick. The departmental state physician in turn complained that it was impossible to fight an epidemic with the funds available, barely 750 soles, when the cost was estimated at 33 600 soles just for wire frames and mosquito netting.[76]

Finally, in August 1933 the Ministry of Development allotted 30 000 soles to fight malaria in Cuzco, and sent Eleodoro A. Camacho, an important official in the Ministry with other physicians to inspect the area.[77] In Cuzco, Camacho organized a campaign command post with the departmental authorities and the landowners of La Convención and Lares under the direction of the prefect, and moved physicians from other provinces to the area of the outbreak. On his return to Lima, Camacho obtained 100 000 soles more for the campaign. These funds came from the fiscal revenues accruing from the valleys affected by the epidemic. It was likewise established that all provincial taxes were not to be collected, a measure that lasted until 1937.[78]

In other words, an anti-malarial campaign that had the support of Lima was begun only in late 1933, almost a year after the outbreak. The delay demonstrates the concentration of decision-making in Lima, where the sanitation priorities of distant provinces were of little importance. The campaign in La Convención and Lares was a palliative task which boiled down to the sporadic and indiscriminate distribution of quinine and wire screens. The health workers were often popularly known as 'distributors of quinine', because they often did not do much more.[79] Quinine did not reach everyone and the wire screens and mosquito netting were not effective in rural areas where the population was dispersed. Many dwellings were of cane, straw and wood through which the insects passed whether windows and doors were covered or not. The only buildings where wire screening was useful were the few made of adobe bricks or stone. Mosquito netting was likewise used to clothe the children and as a mattress on which to sleep.[80]

According to the doctors, the anti-malarial campaign proved futile partly because, with some exceptions, the landowners did not care about the health of their labourers.[81] In May 1933 Samuel Geller found in Huayopata that all *haciendas* had swampland, no dwellings had wire screens and two of them were abandoned. Apparently only one of the biggest rural estates destroyed swamps and distributed medicines and wire screens. The foreman of another *hacienda* complained that he was being compelled to tend to the sick at the *hacienda*'s expense, but without having received the necessary resources.[82] Desperate because his requests were not being heeded, the manager of Huyro *hacienda* resigned his position in August 1933 because he was needlessly endangering 'his life and that of his family'.[83]

The landowners argued that it was not enough to dry up swamps, and pointed out the losses the epidemic had caused them. According to Carmen Vargas de Romanville, the owner of the Huadquiña *hacienda*, her predicament was unbearable because the peons had died, those who survived malaria had fled, and weeds were infesting the fields.[84] For the landowners it was all the fault of the authorities, who demanded of them tasks which could not be carried out, and of the health workers who worked in a casual way. Criticizing the visit made by Camacho, they declared that he had never been able to observe the epidemic directly, and that 'nine sick men died without being cared for while he [Camacho] was regaled with champagne'.[85]

The clash between the landowners and the authorities surfaced in a charge levied against Geller. According to the landowners, this physician resold the quinine sent from Lima in his pharmacy and in that of his brother, both of which were in Quillabamba. Some residents of this town denounced Geller with the support of the Cuzco Society of Artisans. However, Geller was defended by Sarasola, by the Quillabamba town council and by *El Sol*, a Cuzco newspaper.[86] The charges against him were probably due to resentment over the strict measures he took, to his brief tenure (he had only been state physician since 1930) or to mistrust since he was a foreigner. On the other hand, Geller's financial position might have raised suspicions for he worked six months without a salary, even though this same fact might suggest that he did his duty. The truth of the matter is that quinine became a scarce and expensive commodity in a crisis situation, when it took up to 20 days to arrive from Lima. Pharmacists and some sick individuals who feigned taking the drug and then sold it took advantage of the circumstances. Even more serious was the charge that quinine was being replaced by bicarbonate, starch and *albayalde*, a toxic substance made from lead.[87]

The epidemic also showed popular perceptions and attitudes *vis-à-vis* health and disease.[88] Many refused to take quinine because it was considered a warm beverage with a bitter taste that was of no use against a disease whose very characteristics were heat and a fever. These ideas reflected the persistence of old Indian beliefs combined with Hippocratic notions which said the cure had to apply the opposite of the ailment.[89] Quinine was also rejected because of the disgusting treatment usually applied, which included strong doses of purgatives in the belief that the medicine would have a better effect on an empty stomach. Normal doses were also often applied without considering its collateral effects on undernourished, anaemic or alcoholic patients. This rejection led to attempts to make people take quinine by force.[90]

There was always a lack of communication between the health workers and the people because many physicians did not speak Quechua and considered that the resistance of the landowners and popular Indian beliefs were serious hindrances. According to one of them: 'The human factor is the greatest obstacle for the popularization of hygiene. Most have no faith at all in the progress of medicine.'[91]

Malaria rolled forward in the midst of the inactivity of the landowners, the doubts about the physicians and the resistance of the people, and then died out after eliminating or infecting every susceptible community. At that moment Sarasola described the human landscape of La Convención: 'yellow countenances, anaemic children, young people with signs of premature senility', and peons who could not endure 'one week's work'.[92] His description and other sources indicate that a change in the type of malaria prevalent in the region had taken place. In other words, there was a change from an epidemiological profile marked by *Plasmodium falciparum* to another where *Plasmodium vivax* prevailed, and malaria became less tragic, albeit endemic.

According to official sources, during the epidemic 6000 people died and 15 000 contracted the disease. This was a high figure for a population of 25 000.[93] According to another estimate, between 8000 and 10 000 more died.[94] It is not easy to establish an accurate figure where no adequate public records existed, and where any place could be used to bury the dead. Several studies state the epidemic was a demographic catastrophe which it took years for the region to get over. Another effect of the epidemic was the sale of *haciendas* at rock-bottom prices, thus favouring the concentration of rural holdings.[95]

Years later, the concern over malaria was used to begin sorting out the health problems of the region. Particularly important was the establishment in 1937 of the Cuzco Anti-Malarial Service of the Ministry of Health, which enabled the State to supervise the compliance of landowners with their sanitary obligations, check the illicit sale of quinine and distribute the drug free of charge.[96] The Anti-Malarial Service opened its main office in Quillabamba and was headed by the physician Ricardo Monteagudo, a member of one of the regional landed families. This gave rise to a favourable political milieu for the solution of sanitation deficiencies which was used to advantage by Monteagudo, who demanded that the State provide safe drinking water and sewers, refurbish Quillabamba Hospital, set up dispensaries and carry out sanitation projects.[97]

Migrants returned to La Convención once malaria was controlled. The province grew from 27 243 to 61 901 inhabitants during 1940–60, a growth rate of slightly over 100 per cent due particularly to migration.[98] Control of malaria, new communication routes and the return of the migrants transformed the valley's produce from one of mainly coca, sugar cane and fruit, into a flourishing agricultural economy based on coffee and tea.

The State and malaria

The State centralized its activities to control malaria in Peru shortly after the epidemic in La Convención. As from 1933, the Hygiene and Prophylaxis Service of the Ministry of Health had some support from the National Agrarian Society and was able to study the conditions of malaria transmission and control in Carabayllo. Paz Soldán, the lecturer on hygiene in the University of San Marcos who participated in this effort, headed another important study in the Cañete valley in 1936. The spleen index was used for the first time in Peru both at Carabayllo and Cañete to measure endemicity. This index measured the proportion of individuals with an enlarged spleen, a common reaction to repeated malarial infections.[99]

These two events helped prepare a group which in 1937 became the Technical Department of Malaria within the newly created Ministry of Public Health, Labour and Social Promotion. Campaigns were begun during those years in several regions, malarial hospitals were built, specialized personnel were hired (including engineers) and the National Agrarian Society sold quinine at cost price.[100] Finally, in 1941, the National Anti-Malarial and Rural Health Service was formed as a branch in the Ministry for the prevention of malaria, to assist the people, and to keep records. This was part of the establishment of specialized services. (The branches for tuberculosis and venereal diseases were established at the same time.)[101] The national services gained greater autonomy, staff and budget in 1942, when the Ministry of Public Health, Labour and Social Promotion became the Ministry of Public Health and Social Work. In 1943 copper arsenite was likewise produced locally to substitute Paris green, which was expensive and hard to obtain during the Second World War.[102] This ushered in a second period in the history of malarial control in Peru.

The political context of these transformations was given by the Manuel Prado administration (1939–45), the democratic experiment of Bustamante y Rivero (1945–47) and the military regime of Manuel A. Odría (1948–56). These administrations were marked by their closeness to US interests, the influence of agricultural export sectors (sugar and rice producers), and by populist social policies which extended the coverage of education and health services.[103] This extension crystallized in the establishment of Social Security for Workers in 1936, and Social Security for Employees in 1948, which covered illness, maternity leave, retirement and incapacitation of the workers registered. Some of these administrations made public health a symbol of their legitimacy. The slogan of Odría was 'health, education, and work', and he himself established a National Health and Welfare Fund in 1952 which led to the construction and implementation of hospitals, forestalled transmissible diseases, and supported private welfare societies until the 1970s. The fund later had an important role in the campaign for the eradication of malaria.

During this period the arguments associating the control of malaria with agricultural development gained importance. These arguments stressed the lack of labour, the depreciation of estates due to the presence of swamps or malarial areas, the losses brought about by the fall in individual work performance, and the cost of medical assistance. To this was added a renewed insistence from the military, businessmen, politicians and physicians on developing the tropical forest. The military experienced the significance malaria had for frontier garrisons during the skirmishes with Colombia in 1932, and the war with Ecuador in 1941. The State, politicians and entrepreneurs began to take an interest in the forest, to sponsor its colonization and to protect the health of the settlers.[104] For them, the tropical forest seemed to be an unexplored area, unexploited and profitable. The anti-malarial struggle in the tropical forest was traditionally limited to building dwellings far from the breeding grounds of mosquitoes, to cleaning water tanks and to the use of mosquito netting, but it was generally believed that the control of malaria in this region was impossible or not essential.[105] Physicians like Paz Soldán and Maxime Kuczynski Godard declared that the tropical forest was habitable and profitable if investments were made in sanitation. Their statements stressed the economic losses brought about by malaria, and the need to spend money in the sanitation infrastructure in order to protect first the settlers and, later, the natives. For Kuczynski Godard, 'hygienic control [of the tropical forest] should come before human settlement'.[106] For Paz Soldán, 'without health there is no lasting control of the land'.[107]

The argument for public health as a prerequisite for economic development strengthened the anti-malarial campaign. The budget allocated for this goal grew from 320 662 soles to 1 300 000 between 1938 and 1943, an upward trend that helped to increase personnel and the provision of quinine, to improve anti-malarial hospitals, to send students abroad and to establish eight anti-malarial services in the departments of Lima, Cuzco, and Ayacucho, in the provinces of Cañete, Chancay and Camaná, and in the Moche and Tambo river valleys.[108] In the early 1940s an attempt was also made to prevent 'man-made' malaria, that is, the building of roads and other works were supervised to prevent their giving rise to larval breeding grounds.[109] These measures went hand in hand with regulations on quinine. In a reflection of the tension caused by the Second World War (the US government wanted to protect its soldiers in the Pacific since the Japanese had captured Java, the major quinine producer), the USA and Peru signed agreements prohibiting the export of Peruvian bark, and established a quinine factory.[110]

The anti-malarial campaign in Peru received more US support from the Interamerican Cooperative Public Health Service (Servicio Cooperativo Interamericano de Salud Pública, SCISP) and the Rockefeller Foundation (RF). The SCISP had its origins in a Pan-American conference held in 1942, where several co-operative health programmes were established. The SCISP was set up in the Ministry of Health after a visit from the Director of Sanitation in the Institute of Inter-American Affairs. This service, which managed the economic and technical assistance of the USA and employed up to 750 Peruvians in 1953, worked on a regular basis until the 1960s. In its early years the SCISP worked in the tropical forest and in Chimbote, a port located 400 kilometres north of Lima. For these projects the US government allocated US$1 350 000.[111] Lectures on sanitation were promoted in the tropical forest, and a modern hospital was built in the main Amazon city, Iquitos.

The campaign in the small coastal town of Chimbote was more ambitious as it centred on an integral sanitation approach that would lay the foundations for an industrial and commercial centre. Chimbote had been chosen as the site where Peru's iron and steel industry would be installed. At the time this was considered an essential step for a self-sustained economic development, and was the first step in the development of the fishmeal industry. The work of the SCISP consisted in draining seven swamps covering 887 000 m^2, installing safe drinking water and sewage systems, and building a modern hospital.[112] This work gave precedence to the prevention of malaria, which was not widespread in Chimbote. Haematological tests taken in children showed the rate of malarial infection was low (9 per cent). However, bearing in mind that a massive migration to Chimbote was expected, the officials in charge of the project considered that it was essential that an epidemic be prevented.[113]

Prevention was also at the root of the co-operation between the Peruvian government and the Rockefeller Foundation. During 1941–48 both signed agreements to support the Ministry of Health through donations from the foundation that would gradually diminish, while the contribution made by the Peruvian government was expected to increase.[114] These funds financed the malaria and yellow fever services, the National Institute of Hygiene, the establishment of an exemplary experimental sanitation service in Ica and an attempted eradication of *Anopheles* from the coastal valleys.

The experiment was based on the idea that coastal valleys were so isolated from one another by deserts that they could be considered islands, and so it was possible to eliminate the mosquitoes in one valley only. Lurín was chosen in the hope that the results could be repeated. In March 1943 the application of larvaecides seemed to be successful after less than a year's work, because the presence of mosquitoes was minimal. However, larvae breeding grounds appeared in April of that year, towards the end of the rainy season in the highlands. On the other hand, the cotton harvest attracted new immigrants. The RF closed its activities in Lurín shortly after facing these problems, concluding that the density of mosquitoes could be controlled on the coast, but malaria could not be eradicated.[115]

Despite these results, the RF helped bring to Peru the crucial anti-malarial technical innovation: DDT. This was an insecticide that remained active for months, thus eliminating the need for repeated spraying. The DDT was less expensive than the larvaecides and not only did it cheapen the drive against malaria, it also changed its direction. Once this insecticide was available, the emphasis of the campaign changed from the elimination of larvae to that of adult mosquitoes. In 1946 the RF carried out experiments with DDT in Pisco, significantly reducing the density of mosquitoes. Members of the National Anti-Malarial Service were trained by the RF and began to use DDT in four coastal valleys. With the help of the RF, the service fumigated 16 coastal valleys in 1947.[116]

The experience acquired in the 1940s was essential when enlisting the support of new governmental and private institutions. For example, in 1944 the Social Security Bank (Caja Nacional del Seguro Social) collaborated with the anti-malarial services of Cañete, Chancay and Trujillo, the Peruvian Corporation of the Santa Valley backed the control of malaria in Chimbote and, in 1947, the Empresas Eléctricas Asociadas and Hidroandina S.A. carried out a treatment programme with DDT in Santa Eulalia. In 1953 the areas near roads were sprayed with DDT in 50 valleys (47 on the coast and 3 in the tropical forest).

The DDT initially encouraged the traditional reductionism that regarded sanitation work as a war between mosquitoes and health workers, where the people were a hindrance. Some health workers still believed it was a matter of breaking up the biological transmission, and that the problem lay in the resistance shown by the people. In the words of a health official at the time:

> It is quite deplorable that we still have to struggle against members of our own species, who instead of being our allies are in league with the enemy; veritable 'fifth-columnists' in the war against a disease which is worse

> than any enemy army marching through our frontiers and ravaging our country.[117]

With DDT, the idea that work against malaria was painful and repeated was likewise abandoned, and it was felt that permanent achievements were possible.[118] The relative success of control showed in the fall in the rate of morbidity from malaria per 100 000 inhabitants, from an average of 945 cases a year from 1941 to 1946, to 490 cases from 1947 to 1958.[119] Even more promising was the fact that only 20 000 cases of malaria were reported in 1950, while the number had been 95 349 in 1944. Of the cases registered in 1950, 4311 were from the highlands and made an average of 295 malaria cases per 100 000 inhabitants. That same year there were 13 425 cases on the coast, with a rate of 803 per 100 000 inhabitants, and 2321 cases in the tropical forest, with a rate of 965 per 100 000.[120]

One of the most important effects the control of malaria had was the increase in migrations from the highlands to the coast and to the tropical forest. Migration increased after 1940 due to the confluence of factors like urban growth on the coast, industrialization and a crisis in the highland rural estates. Urban growth was marked wherever an intense anti-malarial campaign took place, as in Chimbote, which grew from 4000 inhabitants in 1946 to 50 000 by 1958.[121] Just as malaria served to consolidate the geographical distribution of Peru's population until the 1940s, so the anti-malarial drive helped to undo this distribution. Because of migration, during 1940–72 Peru changed from a predominantly rural country into one where most people lived in urban centres, and from one where most of its population lived in the highlands to a predominantly coastal one. According to the censuses of 1940, 1961 and 1972, the proportion of rural population was 73 per cent, 60 per cent and 47 per cent, respectively, of the total population, while the growth of the urban segment was 27 per cent, 40 per cent, and 53 per cent, respectively, of Peru's population.[122]

However, spraying with DDT declined towards the mid-1950s even though 3 million Peruvians still lived in areas considered to be at high malarial risk. The significance that the disease still had in Peru is borne out by the fact that from 1946 to 1955 malaria held the first and tenth position as the prime cause of Peru's morbidity and mortality respectively.[123] However, the distribution of malaria began an intriguing evolution. While it decreased at the national level, particularly on the coast, and retained a rate of 128 cases per 100 000 inhabitants, in the highlands it rose to a rate of 143 per 100 000. The tropical forest in turn retained a high rate of morbidity with 852 cases per 100 000 inhabitants; there, malaria was the most important disease after hookworm.[124] This development was due to the increase in migration to and from the highlands to the coast and the tropical forest.

The rise and fall of eradication

The drive against malaria received a new impulse in Peru in the late 1950s, when the most important campaign in terms of its scope, resources and results, was organized. This campaign, which had the 'eradication of malaria in all of the national territory in the least time possible' as its goal, was begun in 1957 thanks to the support of the Pan American Health Organization and the United Nations Children's Fund (UNICEF).[125] An agreement signed by the Peruvian government stipulated that Peru would supply the personnel (organized into a National Service for the Eradication of Malaria) and the financial resources through a special government fund that the Ministry of Health sponsored (the Fondo Nacional de Salud y Bienestar Social). For its part, UNICEF provided the vehicles, equipment, insecticide and some medications. The Pan American Health Organization contributed technical assistance, trained the personnel and supplied medicines. The agreement was sponsored by a visit to Lima of Fred Soper, a former official in the RF who was then head of the Pan American Health Office and who had masterminded eradication. Soper insisted that the government's efforts were part of a world-wide drive against the major problem of the American continent, much like Hanson's and the Rockefeller's public relations campaign against yellow fever in the 1920s, albeit with more success.[126]

The decision to eradicate malaria in Peru was part of an international sanitation project which was convinced it would attain its goal. It was believed that five years of consistent work with insecticide and medicines would be successful and more convenient than unlimited expenditures on the endless task of controlling the disease. Finally, it was considered that other diseases would also be controlled with the campaign (DDT eliminated the vectors of murine typhus, yellow fever and dengue) and the health services would come out strengthened. Eradication was framed within the development model of the time, which entailed leaving behind the export model, the establishment of import-substitution industries and the modernization of agriculture. These objectives required the development of a stable labour force in the cities which could undergo intense work.

The campaign was organized in four precise and successive stages which were impressive for their organization and cohesion.[127] The first, or preparatory phase lasted for a year, and consisted in the delimitation of the work area, the training of personnel and the establishment of checkpoints. The second, or attack phase, lasted four years and consisted in the semestral application of DDT to dwellings plus the administering of medicines until transmission was broken. The results obtained were concurrently appraised with blood samples taken at the checkpoints. The third, or consolidation phase, which lasted between one and three years, began when the breakdown of transmission was attained with the elimination of adult mosquitoes and their breeding grounds, and all those ill were treated. The application of insecticide was suspended in this phase, while the health workers turned their attention to an epidemiological watch and to the identification and treatment of unexpected cases. The fourth and last stage, which was known as the phase of follow-up, was used to confirm the absence of malaria and to declare its eradication. Unlike the others, this stage was carried out by the regular health services.

The campaign began in November 1957 with 67 633 applications of insecticide on the coast. From 1959 to1962 these were not less than 600 000 a year in all five of the areas the country was divided into. Another sign of the magnitude of the task was the increase in the staff of the service from 568 in 1957 to 820 in 1962. The budget of the programme rose from 14 022 978 soles in 1957 to 28 000 000 in 1965.[128] Logistics were enormous. For example, in 1965 2 million people had to be supervised in consolidation areas, and in the attack areas there were 1.5 million inhabitants to work with.

An important feature of the campaign was the emphasis it gave to the nationalist significance of sanitation work, to the improvement of the epidemiological record, to health education and to establishing a good rapport with the people. These measures coexisted with more traditional regulations like fines and bounties for every case reported. The training of the people in charge stressed the national and professional 'prestige' eradication would bring. An attempt was also made to prevent health workers from committing abuses or thefts, and charging undue payments for a service that was free.[129] A pamphlet entitled *What Every Sprayer Must Know* cautioned patience, honesty and dialogue. It also warned against the counterproductive result of threats: 'the technique will fail unless public health workers are convinced of the need to bear in mind the concepts, the needs, and the interests of the people'.[130]

The overwhelming magnitude of the task was evident in the tropical forest. Almost nothing was known of the Amazon tribes who were spread about in ten linguistic groups, and numbered some 70 000. The work was carried out by bilingual teachers and health personnel, who travelled over many rivers visiting several Indian tribes in rafts and motorboats to take blood samples and identify those sick with malaria. Perhaps this was the origin of the rumour circulating in 1958 that a monster, half-white man and half-vampire, took the blood of the people of the tropical forest. This scared the Campa tribes. However, the confidence of the people was won anew with the help of the teachers.[131]

The major achievement of the campaign begun in 1957 was that it managed to break transmission in several departments. The campaign also intensified the fall in the rate of morbidity felt since the 1940s. Malaria declined from 1960 to 1963. Between 1964 and 1968 it tended to remain stationary but with some rallies (in 1965 in the north coast, after some heavy rains, and in 1967 in the highland valleys). In 1962 the Malaria Eradication Service was incorporated into the Special Public Health Service. In 1965 22 provinces in Piura, Tumbes, La Libertad, Ica, Callao, Arequipa and Huancavelica were three years or more into the phase of consolidation. The greatest achievement came in the late 1960s with the breakdown in transmission in almost all of the coast, in a great part of the highland valleys and in the southern tropical forest. In 1968 the area infected had fallen by 86 per cent.[132] Most of the cases were confined to the north coast, and were of the so-called 'benign' malaria (*Plasmodium vivax* and *malariae*). The optimism of the time is reflected in the title of a thesis: 'A Vanishing Disease: Malaria'.[133]

However, success proved ephemeral. After 1970 the process of contraction of the malarial area reverted, the number of cases increased and the resources available to combat malaria diminished. Eradication began to slow down at a world-wide level. The USA had supplied more than 80 per cent of the funds for the campaign from 1956 to 1963, but it practically suspended its support after 1963 when there was a change of administration.[134] A decisive technical factor in the loss of popularity of eradication was that by the early 1970s cloroquinine no longer gave protection against *falciparum*, the deadliest of the parasites. Even more important was disillusion with DDT. Specialists noted that the mosquitoes became resistant to the insecticide, which some of them apparently already knew at the outset of the campaign, and that *Anopheles* females rested outside the houses, where DDT did not reach them.[135] The DDT was likewise blamed for polluting the environment, food and kitchen utensils. The production of insecticides fell once eradication was seen as a hard goal to attain, just at the moment when a move to stronger but more expensive insecticides was being requested.[136] This was compounded by the fact that the price of DDT, whose manufacture includes petroleum, rose considerably after the 1974 international fuel crisis.

At the national level there were social, financial and political problems. The co-operation of the people could not be retained when the goals were not met at the expected deadlines. This weakened the health services, raised the cost of eradication and increased the gap between research and epidemiological vigilance. As a result, the campaign at times ended as a desperate race or a sceptical routine of little epidemiological relevance. The goal of eradicating malaria lost favour with the reformist military regime begun by Juan Velasco Alvarado in 1968. The administration believed the solution to rural poverty would not come with public health but from an agrarian reform that redistributed land. The government also began huge works that fostered malaria. For instance, migrant workers were housed in temporary habitations built near artificial lagoons in the dams of Piura, the Mantaro hydroelectric plant, the North-Peru oil pipeline and the oil wells in Loreto and Madre de Dios. A new generation of coastal inhabitants grew up without the immunity of their forefathers.

With gold mining in Madre de Dios and the increase in rice plantations in San Martín and Junín came a massive and disorganized displacement of susceptible populations from the Andes to the tropical forest.[137] This renewed the conditions present at the turn of the century, when migrations moved labourers to malarial areas and these were then sent back to their homeland, sick. Apparently there always were endemic pockets on the coast and in the northern tropical forest which reinfected the rest of Peru. This led to the disappointing conviction that Peru's ecology had uncontrollable malarial conditions. There was no structured control programme in the 1980s, and by the early 1990s malaria had spread all over Peru.

Conclusion

At present, the campaign against malaria is aimed at treating the sick and to reducing transmission, but little or nothing is done as regards the removal of the social and ecological factors that reinforce the disease. Not only have the dreams of eradicating malaria vanished, so have those of controlling it. Peru has gone back to a similar condition, albeit not as serious, as the one present at the beginning of the twentieth century. Every day more Peruvians resign themselves to accepting malaria as an unavoidable part of life from which there is no escape.

Perhaps it was a mistake to concentrate on one disease when international experience suggested that control was enough, and that it was only sustainable in unison with economic development. However, the drive for eradication had the virtue of emphasizing prevention. Malaria was long considered a natural fact of life, and the lack of epidemics an acceptable state of collective health. An endemic disease almost vanished with the campaign, and public health began to mean the non-existence of endemic diseases and epidemics. The failure of eradication paved the way for a change in the social and political perceptions, for which the eradication of a disease seemed to be a luxury. The cholera outbreak showed how significant this transformation was.

Notes

1. The fourth form of the parasite is *ovale. Plasmodium* multiplies in the liver and in the bloodstream, releasing toxins that destroy the red globules and cause fevers and shivering. The parasites were discovered in 1880 and their transmission by mosquitoes in 1898. G. Harrison, *Mosquitoes, Malaria and Man: A History of the Hostilities since 1880*, E.P. Dalton, New York, 1978; J. Zulueta, 'Malaria and Ecosystems: from Prehistory to Posteradication', *Parrasitologia*, **36**, 1994, pp. 7–15.
2. An alternative classification is in Javier Pulgar Vidal, *Geografía del Perú, las ocho regiones naturales*, Peisa, Lima, 1987.
3. José A. Estrada Ancajima, 'La agricultura en la costa', pp. 15–30, and Hugo Villachica, 'La agricultura en la selva peruana', both in Marc Dourojeanni (ed.),

Gran Geografía del Perú (5 vols), Manfer-Juan Mejía Baca, Lima, 1986, 5, pp. 51–96.

4. Manuel Acosta, 'Niveles básicos de susceptibilidad del *Anopheles Pseudopunctipennis* al DDT y al Dieldrin en la región occidental del Perú', *Revista de Medicina Experimental*, **12**, 1958, pp. 99–106.
5. C.V. Brown and G.J. Nossal, 'Malaria, Yesterday, Today and Tomorrow', *Perspectives in Biology and Medicine*, **20**, 1, 1986, pp. 65–76.
6. The highest altitude an *Anopheles* larvae has been found in Peru is 2400 metres. Raymond Shannon, 'Observaciones sobre el *Anopheles Pseudopunctipennis* en el Perú', *Revista de la Sanidad Militar*, **3**, 1930, pp. 11–33; Lewis Hackett, 'The Malaria of the Andean Region of South America', *Revista del Instituto de Salubridad y Enfermedades Tropicales*, **6**, 4, 1945, pp. 239–52.
7. Malaria was spread all over the coast. For instance, 24 per cent out of 204 304 patients in the two most important hospitals in Lima – Santa Ana and Dos de Mayo – were sick with malaria during 1900–08. Abel Olaechea, 'Antecedentes de la ley de profilaxia del paludismo', *Boletín de Salubridad Pública*, 1917, p. 17.
8. Pedro Weiss, Héctor Rojas and Alberto Guzmán Barrón, *Informe presentado por la comisión organizada por la Dirección de Salubridad para estudiar la región del Madre de Dios*, Imp. Americana, Lima, 1924.
9. 'Labor del Servicio Nacional Antimalárico', *Boletín de la Dirección de Salubridad Pública*, 1944, p. 157. Rice cultivation requires peasants to work 'long hours with the water to their waist, enduring the sting of the mosquitoes', *El Deber* (*ED*), 11 September 1913, p. 13.
10. According to one physician, 'the strong survive ... and reach adolescence visibly immunized', Alberto Barton, *La Lucha contra el paludismo*, El Congreso Nacional de Medicina, Lima, 1927, p. 4.
11. Maxime Kuczynski Godard, *El Departamento de Amazonas, algunas observaciones médico sociales*, Imp. Americana, Lima, 1940, p. 64; Jorge Chiriboga and Rafael Donayre, *Epidemiología en los Andes y el problema de las migraciones humanas*, Dirección de Salubridad Pública, Lima, 1948, p. 26.
12. *Las Enfermedades transmisibles en el Perú, 1956*, Ministerio de Salud Pública y Asistencia Social y Servicio Cooperativo Interamericano de Salud Pública, Lima, 1957, p. 7.
13. José Gómez Cumpa and Inés Bazán, *Capitalismo y región en Lambayeque, 1879–1930*, Naylamp, Chiclayo, 1981, p. 1.
14. César Heredia, 'Endemoepidemiología de una enfermedad evanescente', Bachelor thesis, Universidad Nacional Mayor de San Marcos, 1960, p. 12.
15. The migrant Indians in a rural estate in Cañete lived apart from the 'coastal' workers in miserable conditions. Carlos Enrique Paz Soldán, *El Malarigenismo del valle de Cañete*, La Reforma Médica, Lima, 1936, p. 32.
16. For example Luis Pesce, *Indigenismo e inmigrantes en el Perú*, Imp. de la Opinión Nacional, Lima, 1906; Germán Stiglich, *Geografía comentada del Perú*, Sanmartí, Lima, 1913; Oscar Miró Quesada, *Elementos de geografía científica del Perú*, El Comercio, Lima, 1919; Sebastián Lorente and Raúl Flores, *Estudios sobre Geografía Médica y Patología del Perú*, Imp. Americana, Lima, 1925; Guillermo Almenara Irigoyen, *La racionalización de la salubridad pública*, Imp. Torres Aguirre, Lima, 1932, p. 39.
17. For some army physicians, the relationship between race and disease encompassed other ailments, too, like tuberculosis, which ravaged highland recruits stationed on the coast. José Alván, 'Sanatorio militar para tuberculosos de la III y IV Divisiones', *Revista de Sanidad Militar*, **5**, 1932, pp. 82–6.

18. Francisco Graña, *La población del Perú a través de la historia*, Imp. Torres Aguirre, Lima, 1940, p. 17. The speech was read in 1916. 'La organización de los servicios sanitarios en el Perú', *Boletín de la Dirección de Salubridad Públicas*, 1927, p. 33.
19. Pedro Weiss, 'Geografía de las Enfermedades en el Perú en relación con las zonas climáticas', in *Conferencias de Ciencias Antropológicas, Actas, y Trabajos*, 140–67, Universidad de San Marcos, Lima, 1951, pp. 4, 140–67.
20. Cited in Carlos Enrique Paz Soldán, 'El saneamiento rural de la costa peruana', *La Reforma Médica*, **5**, 1919, p. 80.
21. 'Memoria del médico titular de Lambayeque', *Registro Oficial de Fomento 1916*, pp. 328–50, cited in Gómez Cumpa and Bazán, *Capitalismo y región*, pp. 41 and 46.
22. Félix Torrealva, 'Algunas observaciones sobre el paludismo en Ica', *Revista de la Sanidad de la Policía*, **2**, 1942, pp. 14–15.
23. 'Sobre una encuesta iniciada para conocer la epidemiología nacional, Yungay', *Boletín de la Dirección de Salubridad Pública*, 1918, p. 351.
24. C.O. Villanueva, 'Memoria del Médico Titular de Cajamarca, 1915', *Registro Oficial de Fomento, 1916*, pp. 247–54 cited in Gómez Cumpa and Bazán, *Capitalismo y región*, p. 64.
25. Enrique López Albújar, *Los caballeros del delito. Estudio criminológico del bandolerismo en algunos departamentos del Perú*, Impresiones y Publicidad, Lima, 1936, p. 116. For a physician, typhus lice too acted like the malarial 'zancudo' in the highlands. Carlos Enrique Paz Soldán, *La Región Cuzco-Puno, estudio médico militar*, Servicio Geográfico del Ejército, Lima, 1913, p. 7.
26. Zszyslaw Szymonski, *Enfermedades Tropicales*, Azángaro, Lima, 1936, p. 10. For people living with mosquitoes see López Albújar, *Los caballeros*, p. 116.
27. For the 'valley disease' (*mal del valle*) see Hermilio Valdizán and Héctor Maldonado, *La Medicina popular peruana* (3 vols), Imp. Torres Aguirre, Lima, 1922, p. 267; 'La organización de los servicios', p. 33.
28. Cited by Gómez Cumpa and Bazán, *Capitalismo y región*, p. 63.
29. Zoila Mendoza-Walker, interview, 21 June 1989.
30. Lucio D. Castro, 'El Chujchu, folklore andino', *Perú Indígena*, **4**, 1953, p. 100.
31. Antonello Gerbi, *El Perú en marcha*, Banco Italiano, Lima, 1941, p. 176.
32. 'Paludismo y su profilaxis en Pacasmayo', in *Primeras Jornadas*, p. 323.
33. Servicio Nacional Antimalárico, *La Lucha Antimalárica en el Perú: Leyes, decretos y resoluciones*, Dirección de Salubridad Pública, Lima, 1945, p. 68.
34. Ibid., pp. 40–42.
35. Gerardo Klinge, *Arroz y malaria*, Sociedad Nacional Agraria, Lima, 1932; Gerardo Klinge, *La agricultura de la costa y la situación alimentaria*, Sociedad Nacional Agraria, Lima, 1944.
36. Klinge., *Arroz y malaria*, p. 16.
37. *J. Antonio Escarcena to Prefecto, 22 May 1940*, Serie Prefectura Ayacucho, Subserie Oficios Recibidos, Leg. 98, Years 1915–58, Archivo Departamental de Ayacucho, Ayacucho (ADA).
38. '*Vecinos de Montaña de Acón, 1 September 1941*', and *J. Antonio Escarcena to Prefecto, 7 January 1941*, Serie Prefectura Ayacucho, Subserie Oficios Recibidos, Leg. 98. Years 1915–58, ADA.
39. Weiss, Rojas and Guzmán Barrón, *Informe*, p. 112.
40. Paz Soldán, *Malarigenismo*, p. 35.
41. Raúl Rebagliati, 'La situación epidemiológica del Perú en 1939', *Boletín de la Dirección de Salubridad Pública*, 1940, p. 243.

42. Ezequiel A. Martínez, *La decadencia de la Facultad de Ciencias Médicas durante la administración del Dr. Carlos Villarán*, Imp. Samamé, Lima, 1937, p. 43.
43. Miguel Cortez, 'Epidemia palúdica de los valles de la Convención y Lares', Bachelor thesis, Universidad Nacional Mayor de San Marcos, 1938, p. 5.
44. Eduardo Fioravanti, *Latifundio y sindicalismo agrario en el Perú*, IEP, Lima, 1976, p. 17; J. Brisseau, 'El papel del Cuzco en la colonización de la ceja de montaña y de la montaña', in Marco Aurelio Ugarte Ochoa (ed.), *La Convención, el trabajo y sus luchas sociales*, Amauta, Cuzco, 1983, pp. 15–34.
45. Luis Ugarte and Samuel Geller, 'La Opinión de los médicos sanitarios departamental y titular de La Convención', *La Reforma Médica*, **117**, 1933, p. 512.
46. F. Cuadros, *El Arriendo y la Reforma Agraria en el Cuzco*, H.G. Rosas, Cuzco, 1949.
47. Jorge Chiriboga, *La Malaria en los Valles de 'La Convención', Andes Orientales del Sur del Perú*, Librería Miranda, Lima, 1947, p. 8.
48. Ugarte and Geller, 'La Opinión', p. 512.
49. Eric Hobsbawm, 'A Case of Neofeudalism: La Convención, Perú', *Journal of Latin American Studies*, **1**, 1969, p. 48; Maxime Kuczynski Godard, *Estudios Médicos de la región sur del Perú*, Ministerio de Salud Pública y Asistencia Social, Lima, 1945, p. 79. A complete primary education was imparted in Quillabamba only in 1925, and it was only in 1941 that water and sewage systems were installed. E. Vergara, 'La trayectoria de la educación en la provincia de La Convención', Monografías de la Universidad San Antonio de Abad, 1947, 7, ADCu. Carlos Aragón, 'La malaria en los valles de La Convención y Lares, sector Echerate, 1936–1939', Bachelor thesis, Universidad Nacional Mayor de San Marcos, 1941, pp. 26–7.
50. In 1928 the subprefect of La Convención could not apprehend an escaped convict because the people protected him, and also due to 'the small number of guards available'. *Subprefectura de La Convención to Prefecto, 11 June 1928*, and *Subprefecto Octavio Pacheco to Prefecto, 17 June 1929*. Serie Prefectura Cuzco, Subserie Comunicaciones, Leg. 4, Years 1927–29, ADCu.
51. For Sarasola see José de la Riva Agüero, 'El obispo Sarasola', *Mercurio Peruano*, **206**, 1944, pp. 3–24; Sabas Sarasola, 'Mensaje misionero', *Misiones Dominicanas del Perú*, **72**, 1932, pp. 161–7.
52. 'Manifiesto de las fuerzas vivas de La Convención y Lares', *EC*, 11 September 1933, p. 4.
53. Ibid.; 'Quillabamba es azotada por una epidemia', *El Sol*, Cuzco (*ES*[C]), 8 November 1932, p. 2.
54. 'Correspondencia de La Convención', *ES*(C), 24 November 1932, p. 2.
55. Carlos Enrique Paz Soldán, *La pandemia malárica en los valles cálidos del Cuzco*, Instituto de Medicina Legal, Lima, 1933, p. 7.
56. *Samuel Geller to Prefecto, 14 November 1932*. Serie Prefectura Cuzco, Subserie Comunicaciones, Leg. 7, Year 1932, ADCu; and Ugarte and Geller, 'La Opinión'.
57. Carlos Monge Medrano, 'La epidemia de los valles de La Convención y Lares', *ES*(C), 17 October 1933, p. 2; 'La mortal epidemia de paludismo en La Convención, informaciones del Presidente de la Academia Nacional de Medicina, Carlos Monge', *EC*, 22 September 1933, p. 2; 'El paludismo en La Convención y Lares, opinión de la Academia Nacional de Medicina', *La Crónica Médica*, **50**, 1933, pp. 374–7.
58. Johaness Willie, 'La Fauna anofelina malarígena de las zonas cálidas del Cuzco', *Revista Médica*, **196**, 1934, p. 645; Luis Ángel Ugarte, 'De sanidad, sobre la

epidemia de los valles de La Convención y Lares', *ES*(C), 29 November 1932, p. 2.

59. 'El Paludismo en La Convención', pp. 343–5. In 1946 a physician found that 34.6 per cent of the patients sick with malaria in the Hospital of Quillabamba were infected with *P. falciparum*, and he considered that this same parasite was the predominant one in 1932. Chiriboga, *La Malaria*, p. 19.
60. Ángel Menéndez Rua, *Paso a la civilización obra histórica en la que se estudia el aspecto religioso y su desenvolvimiento en la provincia de La Convención*, Sanmartí, Lima, 1948, p. 251.
61. Ángel Moscoso, 'Arriendos del valle de La Convención', Monografías de la Universidad San Antonio de Abad, 1944, 3, ADCu.
62. Ugarte and Geller, 'La Opinión', p. 526; Willie, 'La Fauna', p. 649. C.F. Martínez, 'Las lluvias del próximo verano y sus posibles consecuencias nacionales', *ES*(C), 1, 13 February 1939.
63. Paz Soldán, *La pandemia*, p. 5.
64. 'Carta del Padre José Pío Aza desde Coribeni a Monseñor Sarasola, 1 November 1932', in Sabas Sarasola, 'Extraña epidemia en la región del Urubamba', *Misiones Dominicanas del Perú*, **74**, 1933, pp. 4–5.
65. Paz Soldán, *La pandemia*, p. 5.
66. 'La verdad sobre el desarrollo del paludismo en el valle de Lares. Una carta de los hacendados', *ES*(C), 21 November 1933, p. 2.
67. *Alcalde de La Convención to Prefecto, Noviembre 24, 1933* and *Arístides Muñoz to Prefecto, 11 February 1933*, Serie Prefectura Cuzco, Subserie Comunicaciones, Leg. 8, Year 1933, ADCu; and *H. Valdéz a Director de Gobierno, 13 December 1933*, Fondo Ministerio del Interior, Serie Prefectura Cuzco, Paquete 331, Year 1933, AGN.
68. *Alcalde de Quillabamba to Prefecto, 27 September 1933*, Serie Prefecturas Cuzco, Subserie Comunicaciones, Leg. 8, Year 1933, ADCu.
69. *H. Miranda to Prefecto, 7 December 1933*, Serie Prefectura Cuzco, Subserie Comunicaciones, Leg. 8, Year 1933, ADCu.
70. '¿Por qué no desaparece el paludismo en los valles de La Convención y Lares?', *ES*(C), 5 January 1933, p. 2; Menéndez Rua, *Paso a la civilización*, p. 258; Sabas Sarasola, 'El Proceso de la epidemia en la región del Urubamba', *Misiones Dominicanas del Perú*, **75**, 1933, pp. 41–7.
71. Sarasola, 'Extraña epidemia', and Menéndez Rua, *Paso a la civilización*, p. 255.
72. Menéndez Rua, *Paso a la civilización*, p. 258.
73. Ibid., p. 259. *Prefecto to Alcalde del Cercado, 27 October 1933*, Leg. 97, Year 1933, Archivo Histórico de la Biblioteca Municipal del Cuzco, Cuzco (AHBMC).
74. 'Zonas palúdicas; se declara como tales la provincia de La Convención y el valle de Lares'; 'Paludismo en La Convención y Lares; fondos para la campaña', in *Prontuario de Legislación Sanitaria del Perú* (4 vols), Imp. Americana, Lima, 1937, 3, pp. 339 and 380.
75. '*Memorandum: Pernicious Malaria in the Montaña Regions, from Dr. Giesecke to Ambassador, 15 July 1933*', R.G. 90, US Public Health Service, Box 37, File 425, NA.
76. Sabas Sarasola, 'De Quillabamba: hacia la desolación', *Misiones Dominicanas del Perú*, **77**, 1933, pp. 121–5. 'Por qué no desaparece el paludismo en La Convención y Lares', *ES*(C), 5 January 1933, p. 2.
77. 'Para combatir el paludismo en el departamento del Cuzco', *ES*(C), 4 August 1933, p. 4.
78. 'Paludismo en La Convención y Lares; fondos para la campaña, Ley 7805', in

Prontuario de Legislación Sanitaria del Perú (4 vols), Imp. Americana, Lima, 1937, 3, p. 402.

79. Rodolfo Calderón, 'La epidemia palúdica en Lares', *ES*(C), 6 November 1933, p. 3.
80. Chiriboga, *La Malaria*, p. 7.
81. Samuel Geller a Sarasola, 25 December 1932, in Menéndez Rua, *Paso a la civilización*, pp. 252–3.
82. *Gerencia (Cuzco) to administrador general (Huyro), 29 November 1932* and *Administrador general (Huyro) to gerente general (Cuzco), 5 September 1933*, Fondo Archivo Agrario, Serie Compañía Agrícola Cuzco Sociedad Anónima, CACSA, Subserie Correspondencia, Leg. 22 and 29, AGN.
83. *Administrador general (Huyro) to gerente general (Cuzco), 1 Agosto 1933*, Fondo Archivo Agrario, Serie Compañía Agrícola Cuzco Sociedad Anónima, CACSA, Subserie Correspondencia, Leg. 22, AGN.
84. This appears in *María viuda de la Torre to Presidente de la Junta, 19 October 1933*. See also *Alejandro Delgado a Presidente de la Junta Revisora de Matrículas de Contribución, 14 October 1933*. See also the *Letters to Presidente de la Junta de Humberto Luglio, 18 November 1933*, and *Javier Sota, 12 October 1933*, Leg. 97, Year 1933, AHBMC.
85. 'La verdad sobre el desarrollo del paludismo', p. 2.
86. 'Intereses generales, El asunto de la venta de quinina en La Convención', *ES*(C), 4 January 1934, p. 2. Ángel Ugarte a Corte Superior de Cuzco y a Prefecto, 16 December 1933. Serie Prefectura Cuzco, Subserie Comunicaciones, Leg. 8, Year 1933, ADCu.
87. Cortez, 'Epidemia palúdica', p. 50.
88. It was, for instance, believed that malaria was transmitted by the fruit from La Convención. 'Más vale precaver', *ES*(C), 2 December 1932, p. 2. *Sanitario Departamental a Alcalde del Cuzco*, 10 December 1932. Leg. 94, Year 1932, AHBMC.
89. Luis Ángel Ugarte, 'De sanidad, sobre la epidemia de los valles de La Convención y Lares', *ES*(C), 29 November 1932, p. 2.
90. *Gerencia (Cuzco) to administrador general (Huyro), 29 November 1932*, Fondo Archivo Agrario, Serie Compañía Agrícola Cuzco Sociedad Anónima, CACSA, Subserie Correspondencia, Leg. 29, AGN.
91. Ugarte and Geller, 'La Opinión', p. 529.
92. Sabas Sarasola, 'Del Urubamba: el paludismo, hacia la normalidad', *Misiones Dominicanas del Perú*, 77, 1933.
93. 'Oficio del Subdirector de Salubridad', *ES*(C), 5 September 1933, p. 2; R. Donayre, 'Contribución al estudio entomológico de la malaria en el Perú, departamento del Cuzco, valle de La Convención', Bachelor thesis, Universidad Nacional Mayor de San Marcos, 1947, p. 7.
94. Mario Luglio, 'Campaña antimalárica en La Convención y Yanatile', Bachelor thesis, Universidad Nacional Mayor de San Marcos, 1950, p. 3.
95. Hobsbawm, 'A Case', pp. 33–4; and Fioravanti, *Latifundio*, pp. 57–8. G. Flórez Muñiz, 'Organización social, religiosa y económica en una hacienda del valle de Lares', Monografías de la Universidad San Antonio de Abad, vol. 2, 1946, ADCu.
96. Barton, *La Lucha contra el paludismo*.
97. 'Servicio antimalárico especial para el departamento del Cuzco', *ES*(C), 1 April 1937, p. 3.
98. Wesley Craig, *From Hacienda to Community: An Analysis of Solidarity and*

Social Change in Peru, Cornell University American Studies Program, Ithaca, 1967, p. 28.

99. Carlos Enrique Paz Soldán, *Una Cruzada patriótica por la salud de los trabajadores del campo, la demostración de asistencia y saneamiento rural del valle de Carabayllo*, Ed. Rímac, Lima, 1933; Carlos Enrique Paz Soldán, *El Malarigenismo del valle de Cañete*, La Reforma Médica, Lima, 1936; Lewis W. Hackett, 'La Medición del bazo en la malaria', *Revista Médica Experimental*, **11**, 1943, p. 305.
100. The Ministry of Health was established in 1935. See 'Creación del Ministerio de Salud Pública, Trabajo y Previsión Social, Ley 8124', *Boletín de la Dirección de Salubridad Pública*, 1935, pp. 3–4; Jorge Madueño, 'El ingeniero y su intervención en el control de la malaria en el país', *Boletín de la Escuela Nacional de Ingenieros*, **22**, 1949, pp. 51–72.
101. Servicio Nacional, *Lucha Antimalárica*; Ministerio de Salud, *Legislación sanitaria, alimentaria, laboral, leyes, decretos, reglamentos y resoluciones*, Talleres de la Comandancis General de Aeronáutica, Lima, 1941.
102. Servicio Nacional Antimalárico, 'Hacia la autarquía en el control de la malaria en el Perú', in *Primeras Jornadas Médico Quirurgicas del Norte del Perú*, Laboratoios ABEEFE, Trujillo, 1945, pp. 264–9.
103. Julio Cotler, *Clases, Estado y Nación en el Perú*, IEP, Lima, 1978, pp. 273–334.
104. See Servicio de Sanidad Militar, *Cartilla de propaganda antipalúdica*, Ministerio de Guerra, Lima, 1928; Servicio de Sanidad Militar, *Campaña contra el paludismo; instrucciones detalladas para la mejor aplicación del plan de lucha contra esta enfermedad*, Ministerio de Guerra, Lima, 1932; Servicio de Sanidad Militar, 'Editorial, factores de cooperación en la conquista sanitaria de la selva', *Revista de Sanidad Militar*, **7**, 1934, pp. 5–8.
105. Shannon, 'Observaciones', p. 18.
106. Maxime Kuczynski Godard, *A Propósito del saneamiento de los valles yungas del Cuzco (La Convención, Lares y Ocobamba)*, Ministerio de Salud Pública y Asistencia Social, Lima, 1946, p. 52; Maxime Kuczynski Godard, *La Vida en la Amazonía peruana, observaciones de un médico*, Librería Internacional del Perú, Lima, 1944; Carlos Enrique Paz Soldán and Maxime Kuczynski Godard, *La Colonia del Perené y sus problemas médico sociales*, La Reforma Médica, Lima, 1939.
107. Carlos Enrique Paz Soldán, *La Peste Verde*, Instituto de Medicina Social, Lima, 1934; Carlos Enrique Paz Soldán, 'El Dominio de la Selva por la medicina social', *Boletín de la Sociedad Geográfica de Lima*, **37**, 1921, pp. 54–6; Carlos Enrique Paz Soldán, *La Selva Peruana, sus pobladores y su colonización en seguridad sanitaria*, Imprenta Lux, Lima, 1939.
108. Constantino Carvallo, *Memoria del Ministro de Salud Pública y Asistencia Social, 1941–1945*, Imp. Torres Aguirre, Lima, 1945, p. xxiii; Enrique Villalobos, 'Servicio Nacional Antimalárico', *Boletín de la Dirección de Salubridad Pública*, 1943, p. 26. For the budget see Porfirio S. de la Cruz, 'Aspectos epidemiológicos actuales de la malaria en el Perú. Control y trabajos iniciales de erradicación', Bachelor thesis, Universidad Nacional Mayor de San Marcos, 1954 and the table 'Presupuesto'.
109. Ministerio de Salud, *Legislación sanitaria laboral*, p. 32; Jorge Madueño, 'La malaria causada por las obras de irrigación', *Boletín de la Escuela Nacional de Ingenieros*, **18**, 1945, pp. 7–16.
110. *Prontuario de Legislación Sanitaria del Perú* (4 vols), Imp. Americana, Lima, 1937, 4, p. 1206.

111. Peru had to give half a million dollars. Edward A. Westphal, 'Servicio cooperativo Interamericano de Salud Pública', *Boletín de la Dirección de Salubridad Pública*, 1943, p. 92; US Department of State, *Publication 2803*, Government Printing Office, Washington, DC, 1947 and *Publication 5400*, Government Printing Office, Washington, DC, 1955. The SCISB built 7 hospitals, 5 health centres, 20 medical posts and 38 sanitary posts during 1942–57. *Informe Anual del Servicio Cooperativo Interamericano de Salud Pública*, Ministerio de Salud Pública y Asistencia Social, Lima, 1957, p. 9.
112. Westphal, 'Servicio cooperativo', p. 96.
113. Edward A.Westphal and Robert K. Horton, 'Malaria control in Chimbote, Peru', *Boletín de la Oficina Sanitaria Panamericana*, **25**, 1946, pp. 796–809.
114. The Foundation contributed US$598 283, and Peru US$809 163. *Contracts between the Peruvian Government and the Rockefeller Foundation, 1941–1945, 1946–1948*; RFA. R.G. 1.2. Series 331, Box 1, Folders 1 and 2, RAC.
115. *The Río de la Plata and Andean Region, 'Annual Report 1944'*, RFA, R.G. 5, Series 3–300, Box 103, RAC.
116. *'Peru', in Río de la Plata and Andean Region, Semmiannual Report, 1946*, Lewis Hackett Collection, Series 4, Box 19. *International Health Board, The Río de la Plata and Andean Region, Annual Report 1948*. R.G. 5. Series 3. Box 104. RAC. Augusto Corradetti, *Bases experimentales para la eliminación de la malaria en la costa del Perú*, Dirección de Salubridad Pública, Lima, 1947.
117. 'Labor del Servicio Nacional', p. 148.
118. According to one official the campaign against malaria was an 'eternal [war], as eternal as [the] species'. 'Labor del Servicio Nacional', p. 153.
119. The service expanded from working in 10 valleys in 1946 to 20 in 1948. Heredia, 'Endemoepidemiología', p. 72. For the budget see Cruz, 'Aspectos epidemiológicos', the table 'Presupuesto'.
120. Faustuo Fernández, 'Endemo-epidemiología de la malaria en el Perú', *Salud y Bienestar Social*, **1**, 1953, pp. 35–6; Luis Vásquez Lapeyre, 'Patología y población indígena del Perú', *Perú Indígena*, **2**, 1952, p. 52.
121. *El Servicio Cooperativo Interamericano de Salud Pública, 15 años de actividad*, Embajada de Estados Unidos en Perú, Lima, 1958, pp. 6 and 15.
122. 'El Fondo Nacional de Salud y Bienstar Social', *Salud y Bienstar Social*, **2**, 1953, p. 16.
123. Leopoldo Cuzquén, 'Epidemiología de la malaria en el Perú', Doctoral thesis, Universidad National Mayor de San Marcos, 1966.
124. 'Cuadro I, Casos declarados y tasas estimadas de enfermedades transmisibles por regiones geográficas, Perú, 1956', in *Las Enfermedades transmisibles*.
125. Servicio Especial del Salud Pública, *Informe Anual de actividades*, SESP, Lima, 1965, p. 101. 'Se declara de necesidad nacional la erradicación de la malaria, Ley 12714, 31 January 1957', in Ministerio de Salud, *Legislación sanitaria peruana sobre alimentos, enfermedades transmisibles, estupefacientes y medicamentos*, Ministerio de Salud, Lima, 1974, pp. 74–5.
126. The eradication of malaria in America was agreed upon in 1950 at a Pan-American Health Conference, but due to lack of funds it was only in 1954 that it began to be implemented. In 1955 the World Health Organization committed its support. 'Director de la Oficina Sanitaria Panamericana firmó convenio con el Perú para la erradicación de la malaria', *EC*, 15 August 1957, p. 9; Saúl Franco Agudelo, *El Paludismo en América Latina*, Universidad de Guadalajara, 1990.
127. See Sócrates Litsios, 'Lucha antipalúdica y servicios epidemiológicos: ¿Hacia una nueva orientación?', *Foro Mundial de la Salud*, **14**, 1993, pp. 45–54.

128. 6 628 700 sprayings were carried out during 1957–74, Cuzquén, 'Epidemiología', p. 11.
129. 'Reglamento para la erradicación de la malaria, Decreto Supremo 113-DGS, 8 September 1958', in Ministerio de Salud, *Legislación sanitaria peruana sobre alimentos, enfermedades transmisibles, estupefacientes y medicamentos*, Ministerio de Salud, Lima, 1974, pp. 74–5, pp. 76–82. *Lo que todo Jefe de sector debe saber.* SCISP and Ministerio de Salud Pública y Asistencia Social, Lima, 1958, p. 3 and *Lo que todo Jefe de brigada debe saber*, SCISP and Ministerio de Salud Pública y Asistencia Social, Lima, 1958, p. 6, Folletos, Oficina de Investigaciones Bibliográficas y Fondos Especiales de la Biblioteca Nacional, Lima (BN).
130. *Lo que todo rociador debe saber*, SCISP and Ministerio de Salud Pública y de Asistencia Social, Lima, 1958, p. 1, Folleto, BN.
131. Eduardo Guillén, 'Algunas experiencias del Servicio Nacional de Erradicación de la Malaria con las tribus de la selva peruana', *Boletín de la Oficina Nacional Panamericana*, **52**, 1962, pp. 143–5.
132. Cuzquén, 'Epidemiología'.
133. Heredia, 'Endemoepidemiología'.
134. José A. Nájera, 'El paludismo y las actividades de la Organización Mundial de la Salud', *Boletín de la Oficina Sanitaria Panamericana*, **111**, 1991; José A. Nájera, 'Control of Tropical Diseases and Socioeconomic Development', *Parassitologia*, **36**, 1994, p. 26.
135. Manuel Acosta, Marcelino Napán and Carmen Villanueva, 'Susceptibilidad y resistencia a los insecticidas de los vectores de malaria en el Perú', *Revista Médica Peruana*, **32**, 1963.
136. Saúl Franco Agudelo, 'El Saldo Rojo de los insecticidas en América Latina a propósito de su utilización contra la malaria', *Revista Centroamericana de Ciencias de la Salud*, **20**, 1978, pp. 35–54.
137. Cuzquén, 'Epidemiología', p. 94.

CHAPTER FIVE

Blaming the Victims: The 1991 Cholera Outbreak

When the cholera epidemic broke out in Peru, a newspaper in Chimbote registered a woman's lament: 'God is tired of looking after us, and now He has removed his hands from us.'[1] Like her, many were convinced that with cholera, Peru was falling into an abyss. The filth, backwardness, misery and overall misfortune associated with the disease magnified the hyperinflation, the terrorism and the collapse of authority which Peru experienced since the 1980s.[2]

In two months, some 15 000 to 20 000 cases of cholera were recorded in Peru; 322 562 Peruvians fell sick in 1991 and 2909 of them died.[3] For a population of 20 million, this meant that slightly over 1 per cent somehow felt the ravages caused by the disease. By late 1991, cholera had extended to 14 countries in Latin America and the Caribbean, which gave a total of 366 017 cases.[4]

Despite the extent of the epidemic, cholera in Peru had a surprisingly low case-fatality rate of less than 1 per cent, even though it was as high as 10 per cent in rural areas and 6 per cent in the Amazon region.[5] These figures were in sharp contrast with those predicted on the basis of experiences elsewhere, and which at the beginning of the outbreak predicted a dramatic mortality of 30–50 per cent.[6] How was this result attained? What did cholera mean for the relationship between the Peruvian State and public health? What responses did the people make, and what were their perceptions? Why did the lack of personal hygiene seem to be the most important cause of the epidemic, and not the precarious conditions of health infrastructure? These are the main questions posed in this chapter.

A country for *Vibrio*

Neglect and decay. These terms, with their connotation of being unable either to improve or to retain the standards previously attained, describe what happened to public health, environmental sanitation, and health services in Peru in the years before the epidemic. Neglect expressed itself in 1991 in an infant mortality rate of 78 per 1000, the third highest in Latin America after Haiti and Bolivia.[7] Diarrhoeal diseases like gastroenteritis, dysentery and typhoid fever, all of which have similar environmental means of transmission to those of cholera, were likewise some of the major causes of retarded growth, malnutrition, and death in children less than a year old; together with respiratory diseases, these were the major causes of infant mortality in children under five.[8] It is vexing to find that from 1965 to1990 Peru had a high mortality rate through diarrhoea in children under five. Only in Nicaragua, Guatemala and Honduras was the rate higher in the region.[9]

The persistence of diarrhoeal diseases indicates the importance of factors connected to the ecology of cholera, like the lack of an adequate supply of safe drinking water, the absence of an adequate system of disposal of excreta and the contamination of food and drink. According to a study made in 1998, only 55 per cent of the population had access to safe drinking water, and 41 per cent to drainage systems. (In rural areas the mean was even lower: 22 per cent and 16 per cent.)[10] Water is a particularly relevant topic for, unlike Africa where food became the major means of transmission, in Peru and Latin America cholera spread through the water used to drink, prepare food, wash clothes and bathe.[11]

Because of the poor division of labour between the municipalities and two ministries, the supply of safe drinking water was at the mercy of arguments and lack of co-ordination between the authorities.[12] The Ministry of Health was in charge (through the DISABAR, the Division of Basic Rural Environmental Sanitation) of supplying safe drinking water and sewage-disposal systems to areas with less than 2000 inhabitants, while the Ministry of Housing was responsible (through the SENAPA, National Water Supply and Sewage Service) for localities with a population of 2000 or more. The SENAPA advised the municipalities and had connections with the water supply and sewage-disposal systems in Lima and Trujillo, the two old firms in the SENAPA that were not exclusively dependent on the municipalities. It is worth pointing out that as far as the water supply was concerned, the priority for many officials was to inaugurate new facilities instead of maintaining and improving those already in existence.

According to studies made in the midst of the epidemic in the cities of Trujillo and Piura (with populations of 534 000 and 306 600, respectively), the water supplied by the municipalities was extracted from wells, some of which were contaminated by the sewers, and were not chlorinated (or were insufficiently so).[13] Thus, being part of the water supply system was not the same as getting clean water. A case in point was Chimbote, where 40 per cent of the population had drinking water but almost 85 per cent drank contaminated water.[14]

Other reasons why water could be contaminated were its low pressure, the frequent breakdowns in the service and its storage in cylinders, buckets, tins, pots and other containers with wide openings which let people put their hands in. These containers were often placed near the bathroom or garbage. The result was that faecal contamination in municipal reservoirs doubled its percentage when water was stored at home. According to one of the studies made, patients in Trujillo showed a relationship between the dispersal of cholera and the use of non-boiled water from these containers. A study made in the Guzmán Barrón Hospital in Chimbote likewise found that only 16 per cent of the patients with cholera drank boiled water and washed their hands before eating and after using the toilet.[15] These conditions produced diarrhoeal diseases and kept the rates of other diseases transmitted through water high, like amebiasis, hepatitis, shigellosis and typhoid fever.[16]

In Callao, 40 per cent of the population drank water contaminated with faecal residues. According to one study, the section of the Rímac River that supplied Callao simply was 'a great sewer'.[17] This designation was because the river was contaminated by domestic and industrial refuse. Conditions were not much better in Metropolitan Lima, which had an estimated total population of 6 459 000 in 1991, and particularly for families in shanty towns, about 1 617 786, who obtained water rather precariously through the urban network of public taps, from water vendors who sold water without any supervision, from wells close to the surface and from brooks.[18] Although La Atarjea, the main water reservoir of the city, used 5 tons of chlorine a day to make the water tolerable, it could not prevent the contamination caused mostly by poor maintenance, intermittent flow, clandestine connections and other flimsy water-supply systems. Water sellers supplied water to 25 per cent of Lima's population, at a much higher price than was paid for it in upper- and middle-class neighbourhoods.[19]

Conditions were alarming as regards the disposal of excreta. The lack of water prevented the refuse being washed away and contributed to the clogging and flooding of the sewers. Lima's sewage emptied into the sea through three channels located on beaches adjacent to the city. This same sea held banks of fish and shellfish used for human consumption. In other parts of Peru, the untreated sewage emptied into rivers, lakes and the sea.

Sewage was also used to water fruits and short-stemmed vegetables (like tomatoes, onions and potatoes) which need a great amount of water and fertilizers. In fact, many agriculturalists were convinced that raw waste water and sewage yielded better agricultural produce and saved spending on fertilizers. It was estimated that almost 4000 hectares of agricultural land in coastal Peru were irrigated with sewage.[20] The consumption of these products became one of the ways in which cholera was transmitted. On the other hand, neither the sewage nor the refuse could be reused because there were almost no waste-stabilization ponds or sanitary dumps. In many cities, open-air dumping places were the method used to eliminate refuse, and conditions worsened before the epidemic. While 60 per cent of refuse was placed in sanitary dumps in Lima in 1988, only 10 per cent was received in them in 1991.[21]

Waste-disposal systems in rural areas were ramshackle, like latrines or the spread of the so-called 'kitty-do' method (dig a hole and bury the faeces). Refuse was cast into the rivers and the contaminated waters were used to wash, drink and cook in these areas, and particularly in the Amazon.[22] At the time of the epidemic, only 56 per cent of homes had a connection to the drinking-water system in Iquitos, the capital city of the Amazonian department of Loreto, and only 51 per cent had sewers connected to the public network.[23]

Pollution was worsened because the cities on the coast underwent a rapid population growth before the 1991 epidemic, due to the arrival of rural migrants fleeing unemployment, the agrarian crisis and terrorist violence. Population growth far outstripped the construction of sanitary infrastructure in these areas. These migrants and other inhabitants of the shanty towns often had to travel a great distance to get to their work, and at noon they bought low-priced and easily eaten food like *ceviche*, which is made with raw fish or shellfish marinated in lemon juice, and drinks. During a working day in a city like Lima, 2 million people eat food prepared by street peddlers in the open air with no access to any hygiene, garbage disposal, safe drinking water or sanitation systems. The beverages most sold in summer had ice in them prepared in unhygienic conditions. A study made in Piura in 1992 showed that 90 per cent of the food sold by street vendors had faecal residues.[24]

According to some authors, biological factors, too, affected the magnitude of the cholera crisis. In Peru there was no natural immunity like in India, where cholera had long been endemic. Besides, there was a high rate of gastritis connected to the *Helicobacter pylori* agent, which is quite common in Peru and which lowers the defences against cholera.[25] On the other hand, people with the O-group blood type usually develop a more serious cholera, and Latin America proportionately has a higher number of people in this group than any other continent. Among middle-class Peruvians, the O+ group is as high as 75 per cent, and 85 per cent in poor groups.[26]

The lack of sanitation so far presented was the result of poverty, recession, the virtual collapse of health services and the contraction in social expenditures made by the Peruvian State. In 1991, the expenditure in health represented only 23.56 per cent of what the State spent on it in 1980.[27] In the 1980s it was estimated that 6 million people, almost a third of the population, had no access to the official health service.[28] The breakdown in services was also due to the economic policy implemented in 1985 by the Alan García administration, which lowered the buying power of salaries and increased unemployment after unleashing a hyperinflation that reached 7600 per cent by 1990. The policies applied by García lowered the per capita income to $997 in 1990 (a fall of 25 per cent from the 1988 level), lowered the international reserves to less than US$105 million and heightened Peru's isolation from foreign loans.[29] The ensuing stabilization policies applied by the Fujimori administration in late 1990 were harsh. These measures worsened the condition of the poor and swelled their ranks in a country characterized by an uneven concentration of income, unemployment and the absence of a safety net.

The water and health programmes based on these loans did not have access to funds from the World Bank, nor the Inter-American Development Bank or any other international credit institution. Even worse, the disbursement of loans already approved for the improvement of water and sewers in Lima was suspended by these international organizations.[30] As regards the breakdown in services and the pollution in Peru before the epidemic, the US International Development Agency (in Spanish, AID), declared that cholera was 'a disaster waiting to happen'.[31]

The march of the epidemic

In late 1991, cholera struck the coastal population of Peru hard and swiftly. As in all epidemics, it is not known exactly where the first case appeared, but everything seems to indicate that the outbreak began in the neighbourhood of La Candelaria, in Chancay. Between 23 and 29 January, 11 cases of sick people stricken with severe diarrhoea, vomiting and cramps were recorded in the city of Chancay, with a population of about 75 000 some 60 kilometres north of Lima, and were at first ascribed to intoxication.[32] It is worth pointing out that members of the General Office of Epidemiology and the Field Training Programme of the Ministry of Health were in the area by the 30 January.

In the following days, the analysis made in the laboratories of the National Health Institute and the University Cayetano Heredia of Lima identified a bacteria in patients' stools: *Vibrio cholerae* 01, serotype Inaba, biotype El Tor. The Naval Medical Centre of Lima also identified the *Vibrio*. Shortly afterwards, the Centre for Transmissible Disease Control in Atlanta confirmed the identification.[33] The disease was characterized by a watery diarrhoea that began without any pain or fever, but was rapidly followed by severe abdominal pains, numbness in the legs and constant vomiting. The skin also became turgid (i.e. its texture resembles that of batrachians), the eyes sank and had no tears, the mucous membranes dried up, the patients became thirsty, had severe cramps and had no idea of what was happening to them. Some could lose a significant percentage of their body weight in just a few hours, which led to dehydration, a circulatory collapse and most likely to death if not treated on time.

The analyses made established that the epidemic which arrived at Peru in 1991 was part of the seventh pandemic which broke out in the Celebes Islands in Indonesia in 1961, and appeared later on in Asia, the Middle East, Europe, Oceania and Africa, but not on the American continent.[34] The source of the outbreak was ascribed to an Asian ship that visited several Peruvian ports with crew members who were sick with cholera, and whose depositions were thrown into the sea. It is far more likely that the source lay in a massive contamination of the phytoplancton, fish and shellfish that were near the coast.[35] Although cholera began because of the raw fish and the contaminated shellfish, the most important vehicles for its transmission would have been the drinking water, other contaminated foods and the wrong disposal of sewage.

United States' technicians blamed the Peruvian authorities shortly after the epidemic broke out for not chlorinating the water, which would have protected the people from the bacteria. Non-chlorination was due to negligence and economic limitations. Some officials tried to justify it by blaming a controversial report of the US Environmental Protection Agency (EPA), which stated that chlorination entailed a slight risk of cancer. Most epidemiologists considered the risk was insignificant, and was in any case preferable to exposure to an epidemic. According to the director of the US agency, the Peruvian authorities were aware of the danger which not chlorinating the water entailed, and were 'simply using the EPA position so they could turn around and point the finger at us and say, "well, they told us not to"'.[36]

A marked increase in the number of adults treated for diarrhoea took place in Chimbote, in the Department of Ancash, almost at the same time that cholera appeared in Chancay. There was a population of 310 269 in this important fishing, industrial and steel-producing centre, 96 per cent of whom lived in shanty towns.[37] Chimbote also had a big floating population, that is, many who worked in the city during the week and left at the weekends for nearby towns, where they had their families. These workers lived in appalling environmental conditions. The municipal sanitation services could not cope with the garbage that had to be burned, buried or abandoned. The sewage from this industrial centre and the liquid refuse ejected by the fishing industry were dumped into the sea without any treatment.[38]

The three major hospitals in Chimbote – La Caleta, Social Security, and the Guzmán Barrón Regional Hospital – received 900 patients in the first week of the epidemic, and on average treated 300 cholera patients a day throughout February.[39] According to the Ministry of Health, 19 808 cases were recorded in the department of Ancash (population 983 515), 7490 of whom were hospitalized, and 71 died. This meant an attack rate for the department of two cases for every 100 individuals, while it was of no more than one per 100 in the rest of Peru. However, if we only consider the district of Chimbote we get a higher attack rate: five per every 100 individuals.[40] Most of the sick in Chimbote lived in marginal areas, were over 15 years old and were workers. In an area where the disease was unknown, it was spread by adults with a high mobility who bought food and beverages from street vendors.

After attacking Chancay and Chimbote, cholera then became explosive in the north and central Peruvian coast. Hospitals in Lima, Trujillo, Chiclayo and Piura (the latter almost 1000 kilometres north of Lima) received hundreds of patients every day. The most affected places were army barracks, jails and the poorest and most overcrowded neighbourhoods, as these had the most deplorable systems of water supply and sewage. These factors, compounded by the intense communications between the people of the coast, explain the speed at which the epidemic dispersed. Interestingly, there was a marked gender difference in some cities. For instance, in Lima the incidence of cholera by gender was of 64 per cent for males and 36 per cent for women.[41] This suggests that contagion was higher among those who worked and lunched outside their home, that is, male workers.

By late February, cholera had struck almost all coastal departments and moved on to the highlands. The epidemic was intense in the capital city of the department of Cajamarca, which had a population of 122 100 and was located on the western slopes of the northern Andes, at 2750 metres above sea level.[42] Cholera was brought to Cajamarca by travellers from Chimbote, Trujillo and other coastal areas going for the carnival festival (the most important of its kind in all Peru). Unhygienic habits are commonplace at this festival, like drinking from one glass only, or using the same spoon and fork while eating from a single dish. According to a physician in the hospital of Cajamarca, the emergency room had to increase its capacity from 20 to 180 beds in just a few days.[43] Julio Bardales, the Regional Director of Health made a dramatic call to the authorities to declare all of the department in emergency.[44] The vicious circle connecting the disease, poverty and the lack of resources is illustrated by the fact that the sewers running from Cajamarca Hospital emptied into a river that ran through rural areas where the most serious cases appeared.

The highest mortality in all Peru was reached in Cajamarca because of the strong rural nature and marked poverty of the department, which entailed that most of the population lived far from medical centres. Besides the distance to health centres, roads in Cajamarca were wretched and few were paved.[45] Local governments were likewise weaker in this area, and official medicine was mistrusted for cultural and religious reasons.[46] The latter was not just because of traditional medicine, but also due to the growing importance of some religious groups who resisted the health measures taken. On the other hand, the rites connected with wakes, which last from two to five days, had an important role in the spread of cholera throughout the department and in other Andean areas, so they must be briefly described. The corpse is washed the first day. It is not unusual for it to free its sphincter, and it is not uncommon either to have food prepared for relatives and guests in the very vessel used to wash the deceased.

The epidemic reached the Amazon towards the end of the first week of March. This delay enabled a better preparation of the health personnel and the population.[47] The disease spread through the intake of non-boiled river water, unwashed fruit and vegetables, and the cold rice of the popular 'Juanes' (a typical dish in this area).[48] Economic factors like the problems of refrigerating food contributed to this consumption. Cholera spread in many cities of the Amazon forest thanks to the high degree of pollution in the rivers that supplied the people with water. Iquitos, on the left bank of the Amazon River, had its population spread into three big belts: the downtown area, the neighbourhood of Belén and the shanty town area.[49] The downtown area had water and sewer facilities, and its population had a higher educational and income level than the rest of the city. Belén is an aggregate of ramshackle homes built over posts and rafts, with water closets that empty straight into the river. In its main square there is a busy market of agricultural and animal products somewhat surprisingly called 'Venice', that eliminates its refuse by emptying it into the river.

All departments in Peru save for Cuzco had recorded the disease eight weeks after the outbreak began. The official count then was 116 883 sick and 833 dead. From the first outbreak to 22 June 1991, the accumulated incidence (the number of cases with regard to total population) for all Peru was 1037.4 per 100 000 people. The magnitude of the rate of infection was higher on the coast but the mortality was more intense in the highlands where fewer sanitary resources existed.[50] On the coast and in the highlands, the decline in new cases respectively began around 9 and 23 March. The drop-off did not begin in the Amazon area until June 1991.

When the epidemic first broke out, the General Office of Epidemiology of the Ministry of Health deemed it was impossible to make a bacteriological examination of each case of diarrhoea. It therefore considered as cholera all cases of acute diarrhoea registered in any of the areas where the disease had been confirmed.[51] Although this broad definition entailed an overcount, it actually was not that high. For instance, 86 per cent of the children and 79 per cent of the adults hospitalized in the Cayetano Heredia Hospital of Piura with diarrhoea were cases of cholera confirmed in the laboratory.[52] The real cases of cholera were certainly less than those recorded as acute diarrhoea, but the over-registration compensated for the cases unknown to the health services. According to a specialist, the number of people infected with *Vibrio cholerae* in Latin America was actually ten times higher than the amount officially recorded.[53] The method used to record the cases of cholera leads to a study of the official and popular responses to the epidemic.

Official and popular campaigns

On 8 February, the administration declared a state of emergency for 120 days in all coastal cities with cholera. At the same time, a US$4 million fund was set up to control the epidemic. The official response was initially marked by the recommendations made by the Ministry of Health. This position was held since August 1990 by the physician Carlos Vidal, a distinguished officer of the Pan American Health Organization.

Vidal was a member of the first cabinet of President Alberto Fujimori, headed by Prime Minister Juan Carlos Hurtado, a Peruvian entrepreneur. Vidal was acquainted with Hurtado because the Prime Minister was the son of the researcher Alberto Hurtado, the founder of Cayetano Heredia, the most renowned medical school in Peru.[54] On taking office, Vidal found a bankrupt health system. Public hospitals were obsolescent and virtually paralysed, without any food, refrigerators or medical supplies. To make things worse, corruption permeated the system from top to bottom. Going over the heads of his own generation, Vidal summoned young physicians to reform the State's participation in health, promote popular participation in health services, establish a new medicine policy stressing the advantages generic medicines had over commercial ones, and to foster equity and the regionalization of health services.[55] The reformist ideas of Vidal won him enemies, like the officials in the Ministry who mistrusted the young officials appointed by the Minister, or the pharmaceutical industry which feared it would lose benefits because of the preference for generic medicines.[56]

The main worry of health officials during the epidemic was to prevent high mortality, as had been caused by cholera in other parts of the world. It was feared that the disease would spread rapidly through the sewers, water and food since most of the bearers were asymptomatic.[57] The strategy followed by the Ministry was therefore to prevent mortality through the expansion of personal hygiene, cleanliness in food and the rapid treatment of patients.

As for the treatment, it was decided not to use a vaccine since its use was not recommended by the World Health Organization, as it only provided incomplete protection and did not prevent slight infections.[58] The best treatment were the rehydration therapies first applied on a large scale in 1971, during the war between India and Pakistan.[59] These therapies were simple, inexpensive and effective for restoring water, salts and electrolytes (like sodium, chloride, bicarbonate and potassium) lost in diarrhoea, which are essential elements for the body. For many Third World physicians, these therapies were an inexpensive solution that substituted for the lack of an adequate sanitary infrastructure. Patients who were not so seriously ill were rehydrated in a day-long treatment with eight litres of serum, and took antibiotics like tetracycline to prevent the dispersal of the *Vibrio*. Fortunately, Peru's paediatricians and officials in the Ministry of Health were well acquainted with these therapies, as they used them to cure children's diarrhoea.

Since 1980, the General Office of Mother and Child Health in the Ministry of Health recommended this technique for light and moderate dehydrations in a *Handbook of Regulations for Oral Rehydration Therapies*. Uriel García, the Minister of Health at the time, later carried out an active campaign for oral rehydration therapies.[60] This system was consolidated in the 1980s with the Oral Rehydration Units – known as UROS – established in the homes of volunteers. Since then, paediatricians had used oral rehydration salts to control child diarrhoea, especially in the summertime. The medicine was prepared at home and was taken orally using pre-packaged mixtures of sugar and salts dissolved in water. These solutions were the best way to control dehydration, but they did not cure nor prevent diseases related to the lack of environmental health.

Somewhat less known in Peru was the method for treating critical cases of cholera when the patients could not drink the salts, as they arrived at the hospital in a state of shock or were vomiting frequently. For them, liquids were administered intravenously for about five days. Peruvian physicians were not used to rehydration through the vein. According to a physician in Chimbote, at first there was some apprehension that overhydration might cause pulmonary oedema and death.[61]

What actually happened was that some died from dehydration. This was initially overcome using a polyelectrolic solution or Ringer's lactate, industrially manufactured mixtures recommended in the literature for critical cases. The Ministry prepared an application protocol recommending that the polyelectrolic solution should be applied intravenously in severe cases of cholera.[62] Unfortunately, this medicine was not always available in pharmacies and hospitals. According to the protocol, when the solution was not available it could be prepared by combining its elements, like sodium bicarbonate and potassium chloride, in the correct proportion. However, preparation was complex, took precious time on which the patient's life sometimes hinged and required rare inputs like bicarbonate. In many hospitals, the polyelectrolic solutions or Ringer's lactate were therefore replaced with saline solutions (that is, sodium chloride) that were inexpensive, available and effective.[63] In fact, one of the medical discoveries made in Peru during the epidemic was that these solutions were enough to control cholera. Sometimes they were injected in both arms and legs to accelerate rehydration.

The prompt application of oral rehydration therapies and local creativeness in using saline solutions explain in part the low mortality of cholera in Peru. The Ministry of Health had been preparing from August 1990 for the typical summer rise in child diarrhoea, and had distributed oral rehydration salts in health centres and sanitary posts. The health centres catered for some 2000 people and were in charge of applying injections and providing basic treatment. Sanitary posts were smaller institutions that supported the health centres. Thus by the time the outbreak began, there already was an essential provision of medicines and personnel trained to fight cholera.[64]

The Ministry arranged for the sick to get free treatment, and formed specialized areas in the hospitals called Cholera Treatment Units. These units had staff who wore aprons and gloves and followed a strict hygiene, beds with a hole in the middle below which there was a bucket with lye where the depositions went in, and their activities were co-ordinated with the emergency staff and the rest of the hospital.[65] The Ministry also laid down three guidelines to prevent cholera from spreading through contaminated water or food. These were, first, boil the water used at home, second, carefully wash all fruits and vegetables and, third, do not eat raw fish or shellfish.[66] This last suggestion was based on studies that identified the *Vibrio* in marine species which lived near the coast and were a popular dish, like mackerel, horse mackerel and some shellfish such as mussels. However, few patients reported having eaten fish one month after the epidemic had begun.[67] This is why it was never possible to ascertain whether the consumption of raw fish was the origin of the epidemic in Peru, or an important route for its diffusion.

International agencies supported the recommendations made by the Ministry and had an active role in the campaign. Both the representative of the Pan American Health Organization (PAHO) in Lima, and the main office of the PAHO in Washington, DC, where a task force of experts was formed, provided aid which included over US$2 million, half of which was for medical supplies and oral rehydration salts. The rest was used in sanitation, education and laboratory backup.[68] The campaign began by the Ministry was likewise supported by the World Health Organization, European countries and the Health Ministers of the Andean Pact, who were joined by other American countries like Chile, Brazil, Cuba and the USA.

At first, the recommendations made by the Ministry of Health were accepted by the people, the media and the authorities, especially the one warning about fish. There was some exaggeration, for the consumption of ice cream, drinks and fish went down almost to zero, and people practically stopped going to the beaches. According to one survey, 75 per cent of Limeños admitted not having eaten fish or *ceviche* during the first month of the epidemic.[69] This increased malnutrition, as fish was an important source of protein for popular sectors, and poultry, the other meat used to replace fish, was not always accessible.

In the provinces, the medical associations, local health authorities, the institutions responsible for the water supply and the municipalities echoed the recommendations made by the Ministry. Local newspapers underlined the need for, and the ways of boiling water, washing hands, using latrines, preparing domestic serum, using lye as an antiseptic, and avoiding fish, shellfish and vegetables.[70] The preparation of domestic serum comprised combining one spoonful of salt and eight of sugar in a litre of boiled water. Several municipalities likewise formed emergency committees that initiated projects which were not directly related to cholera but with old beliefs, like the drainage of lakes and fumigation.[71]

Provincial authorities carried out the official recommendations zealously and with some exaggeration. For instance, the mayor of Trujillo warned the people in his city not to eat *ceviche* nor shellfish; the mayors of Catacaos, Chiclayo and Ferreñafe banned the street sale of food; the Prefect of Lambayeque closed the beaches to holiday makers and a Provincial mayor in Lambayeque strictly prohibited eating fish because it transmitted cholera.[72] Vacationists were also prohibited from using beaches and swimming pools in Trujillo, and the dock used by the fishermen was closed because it did not meet the essential hygienic conditions. At this site 2500 kilograms of fish were seized and burned 'because it was not suitable for human consumption, and because it came from Chimbote'.[73] In several cities, these and other radical measures of control, collection of garbage and disinfection intensified and were acclaimed by the media.[74] In Chiclayo, for example, the Departmental Health Unit fumigated the cars coming from the south, and a prosecutor filed a lawsuit against farmers using sewage to water vegetables, as this was 'a crime against health'.[75]

On the other hand, hospitals received a growing number of patients that was sometimes four times greater than the number of beds and staff available. In several cities, staff had to be taken from other hospital services to look after cholera, some hospitals focused only on patients stricken with the disease, and the physicians requested the help of one relative per patient. According to one physician from Cajamarca hospital, during the epidemic 'all doctors had to forget their original specialty'.[76] The work could be frustrating because the number of cases increased, medicines were used up, electric power and the water supply lasted only for a few hours, and the sewers of hospitals emptied into the sea or rivers.[77]

The hospital connected with the University Cayetano Heredia (located in San Martín de Porres, one of the poorest districts in Lima) illustrates the magnitude of the task at hand. This hospital treated 200 patients a day during the worst period of the outbreak, and prepared and administered 1200 litres of intravenous serum and 1000 litres of oral serum each day.[78] In 1988 only 32 per cent of all cases attended in the emergency of the hospital were acute diarroheal diseases whereas in 1991 89 per cent of the cases of emergency were because of acute diarroheal diseases.[79]

The epidemic was also a learning experience for physicians themselves, since at first it was the clinics who treated the adults with diarrhoea, and unlike paediatricians, they had no experience of rehydration therapies. The epidemic likewise transformed the traditional criteria of clinical assessment used for those who arrived at the emergency room. As the first thing many physicians did on finding a patient in a state of shock was to 'take their pressure or pulse', it often happened that by the time they 'took it, the patient was already a corpse'.[80] The symptoms were gradually easier to identify, and medical responses became faster. Specialized units stationed at the hospital entrance decided if the case was indeed cholera and began the treatment. The long shifts, collective tension and the struggle in the face of adversity united the physicians, patients, nurses, obstetricians, secretaries and other workers in the hospital.

This unity turned into open co-operation between hospitals, and during the outbreak these shared equipment that was scarce. For example, it was sometimes necessary to carry out the dialysis of rehydrated patients who could not urinate. This equipment was almost non-existent in the poorest hospitals, and in normal conditions it was difficult to get in the ones that did have it. However, during the outbreak all that was needed to get the equipment loaned was a phone call.[81] The epidemic likewise helped reappraise the role that hospitals had in health care. Hospitals had been criticized as gargantuan, expensive and inefficient institutions ever since the influence of the movement for primary health care was felt in Peru in the 1970s. Health centres with only the essential services were promoted instead. However, hospitals became control and information centres during the outbreak, both for physicians and for the people.

La Caleta, in Chimbote, was one of the hospitals that faced the most exacting conditions. This hospital received 54 per cent of the cholera patients in the city; it only had 100 beds but managed to take 700 patients in just one day.[82] The hospital was poor. Its toilets were poorly kept, there were not enough mattresses and sheets, plastic bottles cut in half were used as chamber pots, and water was only available for two hours a day. There was no ambulance so the sick came in on tricycles and were laid out on stretchers, benches, stairways and the aisles. The physicians had misgivings for '[n]one really knew what we were up against'.[83] Jorge Ramal, the Director of the hospital, used the scant resources available to the full, and instilled a mystique in his workers.[84] La Caleta stopped receiving other pathologies and focused on cholera, thus becoming a 'war hospital'. The administrative staff left their offices to help the 30 physicians, 25 nurses and 40 technicians who worked in daily, 12-hour shifts. Ramal himself worked as physician, nurse, stretcher-carrier and janitor. Faced with the threat of a country-wide strike of the health sector, Ramal assembled his staff on the patio and addressed them much like a general before battle. With an inaccurate metaphor that achieved its goal of avoiding a strike, he told them that 'just like Napoleon's soldiers in Egypt had been contemplated by four thousand years of antiquity, so the staff of La Caleta was being observed by twenty million Peruvians'.[85]

This type of campaign that used charisma, voluntarism and few resources was extended to other non-governmental institutions like the Catholic Church, the firemen and a host of survival organizations headed by mothers and wives, like the communal kitchens, mothers' clubs and other non-governmental organizations that applied survival strategies based on self-help. The latter had multiplied in the 1980s to feed the people with the least resources. It was estimated in 1991 that 7200 of these organizations looked after 250 000 people in Lima.[86] The campaign connected organizations which had had little previous contact. For instance, in Cajamarca the vigilantes established by the communities to prevent rustling identified the sick, the firemen fumigated their homes and moved them from distant areas to the city, and the members of the protestant Baptist Church worked in the hospital convincing relatives that the dead had to be buried promptly.

Another noteworthy case of popular participation in the drive against cholera took place in the district of Villa El Salvador, the largest shanty town on the outskirts of Lima, with a population of 240 000. Here, grass-roots organizations directed by a self-managed urban community organization known as CUAVES (which had a record of communal participation in health), health officials, the prefecture, municipality, non-governmental organizations and the Church were all on the same wavelength. These institutions formed a command post which established fluid communications with the Ministry of Health, prepared conferences for mothers, organized hygiene campaigns and prepared the people to treat less severe cases of cholera. A similar network was established that began in one of the 109 oral rehydration units (in charge of about 600 health promoters), then came the seven health centres (backed by 200 members of non-governmental organizations). The network ended in the María Auxiliadora Hospital, the one most prepared for intravenous therapies. Fifty-one physicians, 13 nurses and about 50 health professionals took part in this network. Although the prevalence rate in the Departmental Health Unit of Southern Lima, which comprised Villa Salvador, was higher than in the city of Lima itself, the mortality rate was lower.[87]

In this area, the campaign left a lasting impression of the importance that volunteer work has, as well as the right to free treatment for the people when in an emergency, the pride felt in self-help, and individual responsibilities in communal tasks. The epidemic made the people change their expectations *vis-à-vis* health services. In most hospitals these had not been free for some years, but this right reappeared once more with cholera, and the people demanded to be treated free of charge.

Even so, the campaign carried out by the Ministry and grass-roots organizations did not have the support of all of the Fujimori administration. The lack of liaison and interest in some branches of the administration meant that it was not until two and a half months after the outbreak began that the government decided to establish a National Multi-Sectorial Commission for the Campaign against Cholera, with representatives of several ministries. Unfortunately, this commission did not actually function. The campaign against cholera did not have the political leadership that could have transformed it into a national crusade for environmental hygiene.

For the administration, the campaign was far too expensive and it looked as if it could not be financed either with its own resources or with international aid. Besides, high expenditures in public health and other social policies seemed to go against the priorities of the economic policy applied by the government shortly after taking office in July 1990. Fujimori had then abandoned the gradualist approach he had preached during his campaign and espoused many of the economic proposals originally made by Mario Vargas Llosa, his opponent. In August 1990, when introducing the new economic programme Prime Minister Hurtado Miller announced that it aimed to fight hyperinflation through fiscal austerity, the consolidation of exchange rates and the stabilization of prices for the public sector. The programme was applied as a shock to change inflationary expectations and restore credibility in the government's economic policy.

Another reason behind the lack of support in some branches of the administration was that Fujimori himself was never interested in supporting the proposals made by the experts in the campaign against cholera. An official in the Ministry of Health believed Fujimori acted cautiously and parsimoniously because he was worried that his political popularity could be damaged by the epidemic.[88] In the end, Fujimori did not take command of the campaign against the epidemic because his administration was torn by internal contradictions that were intensified by his command style. The son of Japanese migrants, Fujimori was a university professor with next to no political experience who won the 1990 polls as an outsider to Peru's traditional system of political parties. Fujimori's mandate has been marked by authoritarianism and secrecy, and he has often played one minister against the other, perhaps because of his political inexperience, or simply due to his experience in university politics. (Fujimori served as Rector of the Agrarian University.) This affected his management of the cholera crisis and hindered an effective political response to cholera. The result was that Fujimori never launched a campaign against the disease. He did not meet with his cabinet but let each minister work in isolation. This caused clashes between the ministers and it eventually led to the resignation of Prime Minister Hurtado Miller. This resignation left Vidal without an invaluable ally.

The Ministry of Economy was taken over on 15 February 1991 by Carlos Boloña, an Oxonian economist who firmly believed more radical fiscal measures and a programme of neoliberal structural reforms were needed. His proposal comprised a cut in public spending, the liberalization of the exchange rate, the establishment of incentives to lure foreign capital and the privatization of state-owned companies. In this programme, public investment fell sharply and the preventive measures needed to control cholera seemed less important. This was compounded by a political polarization that discouraged the pursuit of agreements due to the economic crisis and to the presence of Shining Path, the Maoist terrorist group.

On the other hand, Fujimori was under pressure from different economic groups of varying importance, who opposed the campaign led by the Ministry of Health and which included the export sector, small farmers, restaurant owners, fishermen, pharmaceutical companies and groups associated with tourism. Fujimori gradually became convinced that the campaign headed by Vidal was creating a negative international image for Peru. For these critics, the recommendation not to eat raw fish was wrong because it increased panic in the people, sensationalism in the press, and alarm in foreign markets.[89] These critiques pointed out that most governments were behaving as if all food from Peru was infected.[90] The members of the Andean Group established severe restrictions on Peruvian exports, and this lasted until late March 1991. Ecuador also banned the purchase of Peruvian foodstuffs, canned fish from Peru was burned in Bolivia, the import of fish and shellfish from Peru was forbidden in Argentina and passengers arriving from Peru were inspected in Paraguay.[91] Another measure taken by these countries was to distinguish the official cases of acute diarrhoea from the bacteriologically verified cases of cholera. In this way the figures for cholera seemed to be smaller than what they must actually have been.[92] Even so, cholera had extended to all other countries in Latin America between late February and November 1991, save for Uruguay and Paraguay.

This meant that many marine or vegetable products from Peru, including canned fish and fish meal, were thrown out because they could not be sold, were sold wholesale at rockbottom price, demanded a bigger investment to guarantee a longer storage, went through a greater number of checks, and were sometimes almost banned in international markets. For the Ministry of Fishing, Peru would lose US$3 million from not exporting 50 000 tons of fish-derived products.[93] According to a more detailed estimate made by Petrera, the overall losses incurred because of cholera could be split into the impact the outbreak had in terms of foreign markets (particularly in regard to tourism, and the export of fish and agricultural products), which came to slightly over US$175 million, and its impact on the home market (fishing for human consumption, the sale of food on the streets, and indirect costs in health and treatment of the sick), which came to US$337 112.[94]

The Minister was criticized and pressures were exerted against Fujimori in the provinces, too. Associations of fishermen in Malabrigo, Huanchaco and Chicama, all ports close to Trujillo, flatly declared they ate raw fish and 'nothing happened' to them.[95] They also blamed the campaign for the unemployment that fishermen faced. The fish and shellfish retailers of Chimbote made a noisy march protesting against the 'demonization of fish' to the cry of 'fish yes, poultry no!'[96] Officials in Chiclayo declared that the recommendations made by the Ministry had been too hasty, and had doomed 'fishermen, retailers, and humble homes that have fish as their only source of animal proteins' to 'more poverty'.[97]

To ease local and international pressure, Fujimori and some members of his cabinet took an irresponsible attitude of denying or hiding the truth. Confident of changing public opinion, Fujimori and the Ministers of Fishing and Agriculture, Félix Canal Torres and Enrique Rossi Link, defiantly ate *ceviche* in front of journalists. Canal Torres sympathized with the fishermen, announced a campaign to foster the consumption of fish, and stated that marine species were not infected.[98] Some rumours have it that the minister fell sick with cholera after one of his visits, and had to be interned in emergency. Reyna and Zapata correctly label the behaviour of the administration during the so-called '*Ceviche* Wars' as schizoid.[99]

In early March, Fujimori invited the foreign press to a dinner prepared with marine products in the 'Costa Verde', one of the best restaurants in Lima. The President then peremptorily denied the fish were infected, and claimed that if people came down with cholera it was due to a lack of hygiene and to conditions of critical poverty that his administration had received from previous governments.[100] Fujimori admitted the fish in the sea off Lima were infected, but pointed out that the same happened in other cities throughout the world. Later, Vidal realized during a meeting of the cabinet that some ministers were holding him responsible for the economic effects of the epidemic. According to his critics, the campaign that his Ministry had prepared was overblown, had been overly hasty as far as fish was concerned, and had provoked fear in the home and foreign markets.[101] Some journals likewise charged him with having counsellors who had once been leftist leaders. He was also accused of being a member of the Human Resources Group of the Pan American Health Organization, which was held to be 'leftist'.[102] In the meeting, Fujimori himself complained the people did not want to eat fish, neither fried nor boiled (as the Ministry recommended). In his defence, Vidal suggested lowering the price of kerosene; this would make it easier to get an essential product for boiling water in the poorest homes. Fujimori initially agreed but – according to Vidal – the Finance Minister opposed it because he believed this would be a privilege that would only benefit cocaine manufacturers. For Vidal, 'we would not have had this kind of argument if Hurtado [had been present]'.[103]

The attitude shown by Fujimori increased the weakness of Vidal's position, already harmed by the departure of Hurtado. Besides, Vidal had already clashed with Boloña because he opposed a cut in the health budget estimated at 10 per cent.[104] Vidal therefore resigned from the cabinet in mid-March 1991.[105] Shortly before his resignation he appeared before a conference held in the Pacífico University on 'Cholera and the Country We Live In'. There he made a brilliant study of the medical, social and international dimensions of the epidemic, emphasized the low mortality rate as one of the major achievements of the campaign, and denounced that the administration and society had not been more involved in it partly because 'the rich do not catch [cholera]'.[106]

The campaign lost its drive with the departure of Vidal, and became more disorganized. Many officials who fostered communal organization in the poorest neighbourhoods, now found themselves isolated and ended resigning from the Ministry. The poorly paid health workers in turn took advantage to demand a better salary. The 19 700 workers and almost 5000 nurses in the Ministry went on strike between 19 March and 22 July 1991.[107] This meant that the major hospitals lowered their emergency service right in the middle of the epidemic.

The lack of support by the central government and the disorganization also surfaced in the provinces, where committees against cholera appeared which were never officially recognized.[108] In Iquitos, a committee headed by representatives from the Amazonía University, shanty-town leaders, health officials and municipalities lasted for no more than a week due to clashes between the prefect and the regional government of Loreto. The regional government of Ancash dismissed the directors of two of the most important hospitals in Chimbote for political reasons, and Luis Bambarén, the bishop of Chimbote, resigned as head of the Special Commission Against Cholera arguing that no resources were being received to fight the epidemic.[109] Popular perceptions of the disease thrived in this moment full of uncertainty.

Filth and shame

Cholera exposed and produced a series of associations, prejudices and stereotypes which went far beyond the biological reality of the disease and combined notions derived from western, domestic and traditional medicine. Of special importance among these perceptions was one spontaneously born and spread by government officials, which suggested there was an individual responsibility in falling sick with cholera, or that to be sick entailed some kind of social inferiority. It was a perception that coexisted together with other, somewhat contradictory ones like resignation in the face of a disease held as inevitable because of poverty and the lack of water.[110] But during the epidemic other, more encouraging proposals were likewise born, which presumed the solution to many problems lay in self-help and volunteer labour within the communities themselves.

These varied and changing perceptions hinged on three topics: the origins of the disease, the causes behind individual infections, and the measures to be taken. The most classic explanation of the origins of the disease ascribed it to heavenly punishment. This belief appeared with more force in rural areas, among the peoples of the Amazon region and in the apocalyptic preaching of some Protestant groups.[111] It is also noteworthy that part of the urban population was incredulous, believing instead that cholera was a government invention meant to make the people forget the economic crisis.[112]

The surprising and unknown (for the majority of the people) nature of cholera marked the first responses to the epidemic. Some of them appealed to traditional medicine to identify a new pathology. In Cajamarca and Iquitos, people 'confused' the epidemic with a state of mind (*cólera* = rage in Spanish) which traditional medicine perceived as liable to turn into a disease that caused headaches and stomach aches, vomiting and diarrhoea. As the epidemic progressed, the people called the symptoms shown by the patients with labels taken from domestic and traditional medicine, like 'they dry up', 'they shrivel' or 'they wither'. These were sometimes combined with the more technical term of 'dehydration', and with the ability to distinguish cholera from other diarrhoeas.[113]

A generalized account had it that cholera was a disease which came from abroad, and which was not to be blamed on Peruvians. According to this account, the cause of the epidemic lay in the crew of a Chinese freighter which had cast its bilge water in the harbours off the Peruvian coast; the bacteria had then quickly contaminated shellfish and fish. The connection between the outbreak and Asians reinvigorated old sanitation prejudices that went back to the plague in the early twentieth century. A popular account ascribed the blame for the epidemic to factors that lay beyond the reach of all Peruvians: the Gulf War, which involved the USA and Iraq, had polluted the air and sea with petroleum.[114] To say the disease had an external origin freed individuals from blame, particularly when a shameful connection was established between cholera and individual uncleanliness. The search for exogenous causes was also a way for the government to avoid solving health problems that were still pending.

Something similar to the perception of the origins of the disease happened with the perception of individual infections. In other words, many did not consider it to be an individual responsibility, and the filth was ascribed to 'others' and to somewhere outside the home. Many felt the public sphere was filthy, while the individual and familial one was not 'dirty' or infectious. To explain the source, external to the home, of the disease, a squatter in a shanty town combined present-day medical notions with nineteenth-century miasmatic beliefs:

> The water we take is far too filthy ... garbage is piling up here, just a step away from us, and the wind itself blows it all our way ... [and] everything begins to putrefy: dead dogs, animals, there everything is thrown in the corner ... there are no sewers, so people relieve themselves in the brook, that brook is a cesspool, with their feet all who pass take the bacteria home, it is believed bacteria come because with their feet, the animals who pass through there bring them.[115]

Other agents usually held responsible for the infection were the street peddlers, the beaches, the fruit eaten away from home, the piles of refuse and the flies. For instance, it was believed the disease came to Villa El Salvador through the workers who ate outside the district during the day and returned at night to sleep. Some believed cholera was a result of a combination of external agents, including the heat and dirt, but particularly the filth.[116] The following testimonies, from patients in Chimbote, illustrate the perception of the disease as an exogenous agent to the home: 'after bathing in the beach ... with other members of my family we ate a watermelon and had *chicha morada* (a drink made from maize). Shortly afterwards I felt like throwing up and had diarrhoea'; 'on Thursday I ate a mango and on Friday I had a glass of juice in the street ... and a few hours later I was vomiting'.[117]

During the epidemic the administration, the media, the more affluent social classes and even those with fewer resources than the rich, insisted that the major cause of contagion was the lack of personal hygiene. This was held to be the result of carelessness, ignorance, laziness, indolence, and – up to a point – poverty. In this way, expressions like cholera is the disease of 'dirt', of the 'filthy' and 'vile' spread.[118] Some of the symptoms of the disease, like diarrhoea, vomiting and sweating, were stressed to confirm the truth of these assertions. The pejorative connection between filth and the disease was deeply felt in marginal areas, where many denied having cholera when they came down with it.

In late 1991, just over half the people polled in a group of asymptomatic patients (non-serious cases) in Lima denied having had cholera.[119] According to a woman from a shanty town, the denial was because many were 'ashamed'.[120] This feeling of shame partially explains why many of the sick delayed or avoided going to the health centres, for these were located in public areas. Some preferred domestic serums, or discretely visited folk-healers.[121]

The connection between filth and the disease made being sick with cholera proof not just of being poor, but also of being socially undesirable. The connection between filth, immorality and social inferiority could take on a perverse sense wherein filth was considered unavoidable because it was in the nature of people who wanted to break rules that they were well aware of. These people were presented as indolent, disobedient and lazy individuals who particularly relished living in disorder.

The administration used individual uncleanliness to explain the epidemic, thus diminishing the importance of the deficiencies in health infrastructure and also blaming cholera on individuals. This discourse was ultimately based on the old trick of blaming a social evil on its victims. Furthermore, the emphasis laid on filth was due in part to the government's response to cholera. Since the administration could not – or did not want to – employ a solution that entailed improving environmental conditions, the campaign mainly focused instead on preventive hygienic recommendations and in the early control of cases.

According to the discourse of the official campaign the administration sponsored, the most important thing was to change habits of personal hygiene and to improve the treatment given to patients (rapidly rehydrating them at home, or taking the most severe cases to the hospitals). The success of these measures greatly depended on individual behaviour and not on transforming the level of environmental pollution people lived in. The connection between individual filth and the epidemic was thus a way of endorsing a campaign that was not too expensive – and had a lower cost – as one that entailed solving the structural problems that gave rise to the epidemic.

This hygienic approach to the treatment of cholera spread among doctors and patients. Many testimonies show doctors asking the latter what they had eaten. At first they got denials, but the patients admitted under duress having eaten food on the sly from a street peddler, or having been close to someone who was sick. Narrating the disease thus became a kind of confession that confirmed the assumption that a transgression of personal hygiene had caused the epidemic. This served to mark the future behaviour of the patient and was a lesson for those who listened to this experience.[122]

The connection between individual uncleanliness and the epidemic was also sometimes used to pinpoint poverty as the cause of the epidemic. For a newspaper in Chimbote, this was an epidemic 'of poverty' that only thrived 'in filth, which is why it has chosen Peru'.[123] Poverty occasionally proved to be a cause in itself that could be distinguished from all others. In Chimbote, where the image of a noisome city was very strong, a newspaper read: 'Cholera is not the kind of evil that caused the epidemic, but a strong bacterial disease produced by filthy and infected environments.'[124]

Emphasizing poverty entailed a timid critique of the social gaps underlined by the differential lethality shown by the disease. Some held that cholera had a class-content up to a point: 'for ... the owners never fall sick, just the workers'.[125] Others believed the epidemic marked the limits between social groups scattered all over the city because it did not appear 'in, for instance, an upper class district'. Cholera brutally exposed the difference in the urban living conditions of Peruvians. Some lived in a part of the city with safe drinking water and sewers, others – the majority – did not. In Chimbote, the epidemic also exposed the collective contradictions. According to a journalist,

> [cholera] ... has laid bare a ... weak and defenseless Chimbote. Virtually defenseless. Beyond the golden Chimbote, filthy rich with millions of dollars that flow around every day when the catch of fish is abundant ... there is another that has no hospital resources ... that has a population that does not eat, does not wash and has no right to fall sick.[126]

For health officials, the epidemic emphasized the weakness of the health resources the people had been living with for so long. For some of them, this was a matter of individual responsibility, but also of the established order.[127] Part of the people – and sometimes even those who accepted that contagion was produced by a lack of hygiene – considered it was impossible to demand washing hands frequently if there was no adequate water supply. There was a contradiction in terms between broadcasting health guidelines and the ramshackle context of the water and sewer service. A study made in Lima tried to establish whether the infection and mistaken hygienic habits were due to ignorance or to problems in getting water.[128] According to the results, the importance of washing hands was acknowledged but 80 per cent of the water used was infected with faecal residues. The conclusion was that clean water was more important. However, none of these critiques formed an alternative discourse to that of the administration, and the connection between individual filth and cholera persisted.

As regards treatment, there was some opposition to the official methods in connection with domestic and traditional medicine, religion, and habits on the use of water and food. For instance, boiling water went against the beliefs of high altitude communities of Cajamarca.[129] Something similar happened with members of Pentecostal churches, who refused to boil water arguing they could not oppose a heavenly punishment. For many, boiling water was expensive and required time and labour that they did not always have. Besides, many thought boiled or chlorinated water, or water with rehydrating salts, tasted bad and therefore they preferred unboiled water, or serum if they were sick. In marginal areas boiled water was only used for children. There were also some discrepancies with the official methods as regards treatment, for some Indian communities preferred medicinal herbs that cured diarrhoea, like paico (*Chenopodium ambrosioides*).[130] These herbs were used in small communities with liquor and lemon juice, well-known methods of domestic and traditional medicine used against diarrhoeas.[131]

The connection between filth and the disease contributed to dissociate the State and public health in the popular mentality. Deudamia Bautista, a woman born in the poor Andean department of Huancavelica and now living in Chosica, who looked after her daughter sick with cholera in Chosica a town located a few kilometres from Lima, pondered the contradiction between the assumption that the State was responsible for public health and reality: 'I believe there is a law that says we have the right to lead a good life, that each Peruvian has the right to have a good life but we do not, so if one wants to live well he has to find out how to improve his life all by himself.'[132]

The government's work in health was considered more and more as a benevolent aid, which was inevitably insufficient and sporadic. The attitude shown in the face of this was not to demand more services, but to accept and take advantage of what little the government could give. The State was not perceived as an institution that had the task of intervening, nor the people as an agent that had the right to demand. This was not just because the neoliberal discourse considered the government had few social responsibilities, but also because throughout Peru's history, the State has traditionally been an insecure point of reference for the people. The insufficient government aid did not give rise to claims made on the State, as it was not considered capable, or responsible for, health expenditures. The need for protection, the lack of resources and the individual solutions strengthened a fatalist perspective in some groups, who accepted the recurrence of diseases as something natural and unavoidable. According to one dweller of a shanty town: 'Cholera has gone for the time being ... but they say it will come back again ... it comes back later.'[133]

For others, the lack of government leadership presented an opportunity to reinforce confidence in popular self-organization. Campaigns were organized by the people themselves in a few localities like Villa El Salvador, which strengthened the surveillance for diarrhoeal diseases, the lectures on hygiene and the discovery of efficient and cheap methods with which to disinfect water, eliminate human excreta and move food. These measures followed the recommendations made in the official campaign, but also included critiques of its limitations. The leaders of Villa El Salvador questioned the emphasis on the distribution of pamphlets because not all could read, and because there were no material facilities for more hygienic habits. According to these critiques the resources would have been better spent on infrastructure works.[134] However, these critiques coexisted with the dominant hygienic discourse which the official media trumpeted, and they did not manage to crystallize into an alternative sanitary proposal.

Conclusions

According to an US AID report, to control cholera the Peruvian State would have to increase its investment in water and drainage by at least ten times during the following ten years. This entailed an annual investment of US$100–120 million until the year 2000, just to get a supply of safe drinking water for 80 per cent and 50 per cent of the urban and rural population, as well as the establishment of sewers for 75 per cent and 50 per cent of the urban and rural population.[135] This kind of investment was never seriously intended, and cholera became endemic in Peru. In 1992 and 1993, 212 642 and 71 448 cases were respectively recorded.[136]

Paradoxically enough, the campaign against cholera was deemed a success by the administration, officials in the Ministry of Health, and the international agencies. The main argument behind this agreement was the low lethality of the epidemic, which was interpreted as an accomplishment of the medical and sanitary staff. But what really was the legacy of the campaign against cholera? It is not easy to give an answer in absolute terms. The campaign had remarkable humanitarian results from the point of view of healing, saving human lives and providing a hygiene education, particularly considering the lack of resources. This was due to the efforts, the solidarity and the talent of doctors, nurses and sanitary staff who behaved heroically in the face of adversity. It is worth pointing out that for some sectors, like the communal leaders of Villa El Salvador, the campaign was a success because it raised the self-esteem of grass-roots organizations, and because of the support the latter gave to the government.[137] Other gains included a more frequent chlorination of water – it was rarely done before the epidemic – and an improvement in the collection of rubbish and cleanliness in lifestyles and hygiene. However, a study made after the epidemic found that the most important thing for most people was eating properly, and that as far as eating from the street peddlers was concerned it was 'business as usual', that is, things continued just like they were before the epidemic.[138]

An opportunity to improve sanitation infrastructure was lost with cholera. High international officials perceived the opportunity that Peru had let go. According to the director of the PAHO, cholera was the opportunity to 'rouse the conscience of political leaders ... of the importance health has', and to begin 'a long-term action which has as its goal working out a solution to ... the major causes underlying not just cholera but other transmissible diseases too'.[139] However, the circumstances were not taken advantage of by the State nor the sanitary workers, nor did they gender an alternative proposal in non-governmental organizations. The main reason why the State did not commit itself to a greater intervention was the persistence of a sanitary discourse that blames individuals for the disease and gives priority to technical and curative solutions.

The official discourse attained the hegemony despite the contradiction present in the different perceptions of the disease, like that contrasting individual uncleanliness with poverty as a reason for the epidemic. It was partly thanks to this and to its successes in the struggle against terrorism and inflation, that the Fujimori administration retained a high level of popularity in late 1991 and afterwards. In succeeding years, the neoliberal economic policies relegated social ones to second place. Many Peruvians gradually accepted that providing adequate health for the people did not pertain to the State but was rather a matter of individual responsibility, of families, and of non-governmental organizations. It was thus that cholera left behind two conflicting legacies. On the one hand, public health became less important for the State, notwithstanding the generous display of goodwill by doctors and people alike. On the other hand, the crisis presented opportunities for a broader and more active participation of individuals and organizations which peviously had not been so committed to the preservation of health.

Notes

1. '¿Dios nos ha abandonado?', *Diario de Chimbote*, Chimbote (*DC*), 8 February 1991, p. 2.
2. Cholera was first identified in India and became infamous in the nineteenth century, when it extended to Europe and America. J. Snow established in 1854 that it was transmitted mainly through contaminated water supply. This encouraged the clean-up of European cities. In 1884, the German R. Koch identified the bacteria *Vibrio cholerae* as its cause. Cholera vanished from America and Europe in the twentieth century, and took refuge in Africa and Asia. R. Pollitzer, *Cholera*, World Health Organization, Geneva, 1959. According to this author, cholera struck Peru in 1832 and 1869.
3. 'Cholera in the Americas', *Weekly Epidemiological Record, World Health Organization*, **67**, 1992, p. 33; 'La situación del cólera en las Américas', *Boletín Epidemiológico, Organización Panamericana de la Salud*, **15**, 1, 1994, pp. 13–16; Robert Tauxe and Paul Blake, 'Letter from Peru, Epidemic Cholera in Latin America', *Journal of Medical Association*, **267**, 10, 1992, pp. 1388–90.
4. Rubén Suárez and Bonnie Bradford, *The Economic Impact of the Cholera Epidemic in Peru*, Envirolmental Health Project, Washington, DC, 1993, p. 3.
5. Cholera had been found in Peru in 1984 and 1988, but not much attention was paid to it. B.A. Kay and R.B. Sack, '*Vibrio cholerae* Non 01 Isolated from Five People with Diarrhea in Lima', *Lancet*, **28**, 1, 1984, p. 218; and R.A. Batchelor and S.F. Wignall, 'Nontogenic 01 *Vibrio cholerae* in Peru: A Report of Two Cases Associated with Diarrhoea', *Diagnostic Microbiological Infectious Diseases*, **10**, 1988, p. 135.

6. 'La situación', p. 16. Panic broke out due to the prediction made in a British publication, estimating that 4000 Peruvians would die from cholera in April. Cited in José Antonio Iturri, 'A epidemia de cólera no Peru como um evento social. As representacoes das liderancas comunitárias de Villa El Salvador, Lima, 1991', Master thesis, School of Public Health, Fundación Oswaldo Cruz, 1994, p. 26.
7. Programa de las Naciones Unidas para el Desarrollo, *Informe Anual de la Cooperación para el Desarrollo, Perú, 1991*, PNUD, Lima, 1992; and Dieter Zschock, *Health Care in Peru: Resources and Policy*, Westview Press, Boulder, CO, 1988.
8. Amalia Bensimón and Graciela Díaz, 'Factores que influyen en la incidencia de las Enfermedades Diarreicas Agudas (EDA) en niños menores de 1 año, Iquitos', Licenciate thesis, Universidad Nacional de la Amazonía Peruana, 1991.
9. Organización Panamericana de la Salud, *Las condiciones de salud en las Américas, 1994*, Organización Panamericana de la Salud, Publicación Científica 459, Washington, DC, 1994, p. 174.
10. Luis Antonio Loyola, *La epidemia de cólera en el Perú y relación con los problemas de salud ambiental*, Organización Panamericana de la Salud, Lima, 1991, p. 19.
11. R.I. Glass, M. Liberl and A.D. Brandling-Bennet, 'Epidemic Cholera in the Americas', *Science*, **256**, 12 June 1992, pp. 1524–5. According to Seminario, there was 'strong evidence that the major way of transmission was through the water in the public network'. Luis Seminario, Augusto López, Esther Vasques and Marcela Rodríguez, 'Epidemia del cólera en el Perú, vigilancia epidemiológica', *Revista Peruana de Epidemiología*, **4**, 2, 1991, p. 10.
12. Sheila Webb, *Waterborne Diseases in Peru*, The World Bank policy research working papers, Washington, DC, August 1992, p. 2.
13. Richard Webb and Graciela Fernández Baca, *Perú en números 1991, Anuario Estadístico*, Cuánto, Lima, 1991, p. 129. Allen Ries, Duc Vugia, Luis Beingolea et al., 'Cholera in Piura, Peru: A Modern Urban Epidemic', *Journal of Infectious Diseases*, **166**, 6, 1992, pp. 1429–33. David Swerdlow, Eric Mintz, Marcela Rodríguez et al., 'Waterborne Transmission of Epidemic Cholera in Trujillo, Peru: Lessons for a Continent at Risk', *Lancet*, **340**, 1992, pp. 28–32; M. Rodríguez, E. Tejada, L. Seminario et al., 'Epidemia de Cólera en el distrito de Víctor Larco Herrera, Trujillo, La Libertad', *Revista Peruana de Epidemiología*, **4**, 2, 1991, pp. 8–41; E. Vasques, A. Palacios, L. Beingolea et al., 'Epidemia de cólera en Perú: estudio caso-control de Piura', *Revista Peruana de Epidemiología*, **4**, 2, 1991, pp. 47–50.
14. *Salud y los servicios básicos*, Coordinadora de ONGs para el cólera, Chimbote, 1993, p. 23.
15. Luis Urteaga, 'Estudio clínico y epidemiológico del cólera, Hospital Regional Guzmán Barrón, Chimbote, 1991', Master thesis, Universidad Peruana Cayetano Heredia, p. 12.
16. Christoper Anderson, 'Cholera Epidemic Traced to Risk Miscalculation, Cancer Fear Lead to Halting of Chlorination', *Nature*, **354**, 1991, p. 255. In February 1991 it was found that 60 per cent of the water samples taken in non-residential areas of Trujillo were contaminated.
17. María del Carmen Gastañaga, 'Agua y saneamiento básico, Perú, 1991', *Revista Peruana de Epidemiología*, **4**, 2, 1991, p. 70.
18. Webb and Graciela Fernández Baca, *Perú*, pp. 129–30.
19. Joseph Haratani and Donald Hernández, *Cholera in Peru: A Rapid Assessment of*

the Country's Water and Sanitation Infrastructure, USAID Mission to Peru, Washington DC, 1991, p. 16. The cubic metre of water in Lima's shanty towns cost five dollars. In other neighbourhoods it cost 30 cents. Scott Mclellan, 'La muerte como modo de vida: el cólera mata pero la epidemia en el Perú también ha salvado vidas', *CERES, Revista de la FAO*, **24**, 137, 1992, pp. 39–43.

20. Mclellan, 'La muerte', p. 42.
21. Comisión Interinstitucional de Estadísticas del Medio Ambiente, *Perú, Estadísticas del medio ambiente*, Instituto Nacional de Estadística e Informática, Lima, 1993, p. 221.
22. Robert Quick, Rodolfo Vargas, Dafne Moreno et al., 'Epidemic Cholera in the Amazon: The Challenge of Preventing Death', *American Journal of Tropical Medicine and Hygiene*, **48**, 5, 1993, pp. 597–602.
23. Instituto Nacional de Estadística e Informática, *Región Loreto, compendio estadístico, 1991–1992*, Dirección Nacional de Estadísticas Regionales, Lima, 1992, p. 43.
24. Vasques et al., 'Epidemia', pp. 47–50.
25. R. Gilman, Raúl León Barúa and A. Ramírez-Ramos, 'Significado de la infección de la *Campylobacter pylori* en el Perú', *Acta Herediana*, **9**, 1988, pp. 12–16.
26. R.I. Glass, J. Holmgrem, E. Haley et al., 'Predisposition for Cholera of Individuals with O Blood Group: Possible Evolutionary Significance', *American Journal of Epidemiology*, **232**, 1985, pp. 791–6.
27. Felipe Portocarrero and Mario Aguirre, 'El gasto público en salud, Perú: 1980–1992', in Roberto Urrunaga and Juan Julio Wicht (eds), *Informe de coyuntura, evolución de la economía peruana, 1992, segundo semestre*, Univerisdad del pacífico, Lima, 1993, pp. 78–103.
28. Zschock, *Health Care*, p. 4; 'Epidemia del Cólera en el Perú, pautas para su control', *Boletín de la Oficina Sanitaria Panamericana*, **110**, 4, 1991, pp. 277–97.
29. Julio Velarde, 'Macroeconomic Stability and the Prospects for Growth, 1990–1993', in Joseph Tulchin and Gary Baland (eds), *Peru in Crisis, Dictatorship or Democracy*, Woodrow Wilson Center, Washington, DC, 1994, p. 140.
30. A loan of over US$40 million for water and sewers in Lima was suspended by the World Bank in 1986, when only US$12.4 million had been spent. World Bank, *Peru, Lima Water Supply and Severage Project, Loan 2139-PE*, World Bank Report 10230, Washington, DC, 1991.
31. Haratani and Hernández, *Cholera*, p. 27.
32. Seminario, 'Epidemia', pp. 8–10.
33. The serovariety 01 is the only one of the 60 in the serogroup *Vibrio cholerae* that can start an epidemic. See 'Cholera-Peru, 1991', *Morbidity and Mortality Weekly Report, Centers for Disease Control*, **40**, 1991, p. 1232; also 'Cholera-Peru, 1991', for the characteristics of the El Tor biotype and the Inaba serotype.
34. Paul Blake, 'Epidemiology of Cholera in the Americas', *Gastroenterology Clinics of North America*, **22**, 3, 1993, pp. 639–60; Dhiman Barúa and William Greenough (eds), *Cholera*, Plenum Medical, New York, 1992; Leonardo Mata, *El cólera, historia, prevención y control*, Universidad de Costa Rica, San José, 1992.
35. Eduardo Gotuzzo, 'El cólera en el Perú', *Revista Médica Herediana*, **2**, 3, 1991, pp. 105–7.
36. Cited in Anderson, 'Cholera Epidemic'.
37. Webb and Fernández Baca, *Peru*, p. 130; Carmen Tocón and Antonio Acosta, *Con la vida a cuestas, mujer, empleo y condiciones de vida*, Casa de la Mujer, Chimbote, 1994, p. 19.
38. Gustavo Molina, *Salud ocupacional y epidemilogía ambiental en la producción*

manufacturera de acero en Chimbote, Centro Panamericano de Ecología Humana y Salud, Lima, 1982; Armando Mendiburu and María Elena Foronda, *Sondeo epidemiológico de los efectos de la contaminación industrial en Chimbote*, Natura, Chimbote, 1991.

39. 'Epidemia de vómitos y diarreas causa 14 muertos en Chimbote', *Satélite* (*S*), 4 February 1991, p. 1.
40. Urteaga, 'Estudio clínico', pp. 8 and 34.
41. César Hoyos, Jorge Romero and Luis Monteverde, 'Rebrote epidémico del cólera en Lima', *Revista de Gastroenterología Peruana*, **12**, 1992, p. 26.
42. Webb and Fernández Baca, *Perú*, p. 129.
43. Diomedes Mallca Hernández, interview, 18 January 1996. In 1996 he was the Director of the Cajamarca Regional Hospital.
44. 'Cólera: 535 muertos y 90,000 infectados', *Resumen Semanal, Desco* (*RSD*), **14**, 611, 15–21 March 1991, p. 1.
45. Cajamarca is the third most peopled department in Peru. Its rural nature is in contrast with the urbanization of the rest of the country. While Peru experienced a fall in its rurality from 70 per cent to 47 per cent from 1940 to 1981, in Cajamarca it was of only 86 per cent to 80 per cent. In 1987, 70 per cent of the roads in this department were no more than paths, and only 5 per cent were paved. Corporación Departamental de Desarrollo de Cajamarca, *Problemática y perpectivas de desarrollo del departamento de Cajamarca 1983–1985*, CDDC, Lima, 1983, p. 5; Taller de Estudios Fanny Abanto Calle, *Geografía de Cajamarca*, Labrusa, Cajamarca, 1990, p. 77.
46. Andrea Sánchez, Olga Vargas and Isolina Villacorta, 'Actitud de la población en la no utilización del servicio de salud, Llanacora, Cajamarca', Licenciate thesis, Universidad Nacional de Cajamarca, 1987.
47. Eduardo Chuecas, interview, 23 May 1996. In 1996 he was the Director of the Loreto Regional Hospital.
48. O. Mujica, R. Quick, A. Palacios et al., 'Cólera en la selva peruana: factores de riesgo y protección', *Revista Peruana de Epidemiología*, **4**, 2, 1991, pp. 62–9.
49. Javier Vargas, 'Diarrea aguda y estado nutricional en niños menores de 5 años atendidos en el Hospital Regional del Amazonas', Medical thesis, Universidad Nacional de la Amazonía Peruana, 1993, p. 8.
50. 'El cólera', p. 1.
51. Seminario, López, Vasques and Rodríguez, 'Epidemia', p. 9.
52. 'En crítica situación atiende el cólera hospital Cayetano Heredia', *El Tiempo*, Piura (*ET*[P]), 18 March 1991, p. 7.
53. Blake, 'Epidemiology of Cholera', p. 650.
54. A renewable financial fund existed throughout the campaign thanks to the amiable relations between Vidal and Hurtado. 'Cólera: estado de emergencia', *RSD*, **14**, 607, 8–14 February 1991, p. 1.
55. Ministerio de Salud, *Hacia un Sistema Nacional Regionalizado e Integrado de Salud (objetivos, políticas, metas)*, Ministerio de Salud, Lima, 1990.
56. Victor Cuba, interview, 8 January 1996. At the time he was Vice-Minister of Health.
57. L. Puglielli, C. Cattrini, J. Resa et al., 'Symptomless Carriage of *Vibrio Cholera* in Peru', *Lancet*, **339**, 25 April 1992, pp. 1056–7.
58. Vaccination was also discouraged because it gave a false feeling of security and distracted the efforts made in prevention. 'Evaluación de las vacunas contra el cólera', *Boletín Epidemiológico, Organización Panamericana de la Salud*, **12**, 2, 1991, pp. 11–12.

59. Joshua Ruxin, 'Magic Bullet: The History of Oral Rehydration Therapy', *Medical History*, **38**, 1991, pp. 363–97.
60. Flora Macedo and Susana Ríos, 'Efectividad de la terapia de rehidratación oral, Hospital Iquitos', Licenciate thesis, Universidad Nacional de la Amazonía Peruana, 1985; David Swerdlow, M.D. Allen and A. Ries, 'Cholera in the Americas, Guidelines for the Clinician', *Journal of the American Medical Association*, **267**, 11, 1992, pp. 1495–9.
61. Juan Rosado, interview, 15 March 1996. He was then a physician in La Caleta Hospital.
62. Ministry of Health, 'Protocolo de manejo médico de los casos de cólera en establecimientos hospitalarios', 8 February 1991. Documentation supplied by Eduardo Monge. Monge, interview, 18 September 1996. Physician in the Daniel A. Carrión Hospital in Callao.
63. Gotuzzo, 'El cólera', p. 106; J. Cieza, 'Esquema para el manejo de pacientes deshidratados por cólera', *Revista Médica Herediana*, **2**, 1991, pp. 68–9. M. Vargas, L. Huicho, V. Salcedo and E. Monge, 'Use of Isotonic Sodium Chloride in the Early Treatment of Cholera Diarrhea: The Peruvian Experience', *Journal of Wilderness Medicine*, **4**, 1993, pp. 62–7.
64. In 1990 there were 1020 health centres and 3162 sanitary posts in all Peru. Carlos Vidal, 'El cólera en el Perú', *Revista Médica Herediana*, **2**, 1991, pp. 52–3.
65. The measures taken in Ministry of Health. Hospital de Apoyo E.G. Barrón, Chimbote, 'Manual de tratamiento clínico del cólera, Chimbote, mimeo, 1992'; Hospital de Apoyo E.G. Barrón, Chimbote,'Protocolo de manejo médico de los casos de cólera en establecimientos hospitalarios', mimeograph, February 1991, document provided by Eduardo Monge.
66. 'Las recomendaciones del Colegio Médico del Perú', *Expreso*, 6 February 1991, p. 6.
67. Blake, 'Epidemiology of Cholera', p. 648.
68. '27 September 1991, El cólera en América', in Organización Panamericana de la Salud, *XXV Reunión del Consejo Directivo de la Organización Panamericana de la Salud, Actas Resumidas, Septiembre 23–27, 1991*, Organizatión Panamerican de la Salud, Washington, DC, 1991, p. 245. The World Health Organization established a World Task Force Against Cholera. *Actividades de la Organización Mundial de la Salud, 1990–1991*, Organización Mundial de la Salud, Geneva, 1992, p. 107.
69. 'La guerra del ceviche ha terminado', *RSD*, **14**, 611, 15–21 March 1991, p. 5; Bruno Benavides, 'Consumo de alimentos en comedores populares de Lima durante la epidemia de cólera', *Revista Peruana de Epidemiología*, **4**, 2, 1991, pp. 102–8.
70. For instance, 'Comunicado del Colegio Médico del Perú, Consejo Regional de Iquitos', *Kanatari* (*K*), 24 February 1991, p. 5; Dirección Subregional de Salud, 'El cólera puede matar en dos días', *La Industria*, Chiclayo (*LI* [C]), 6 February 1991, p. 3; and the articles in *S*, Municipalidad Provincial de Trujillo, 'Comunicado Público'; Servicio de Agua Potable y Alcantarillado de Trujillo, 'Recomendaciones a nuestros usuarios', and 'Sobre suero casero y uso de lejía orienta el Municipio', 6 and 15 February 1991, pp. 2, 3.
71. 'Consejo creó fondo para la emergencia', 'Acciones de emergencia por el cólera, Castilla', *ET*(P), 10 and 16 February 1991, p. 5.
72. 'Prohiben comer ceviche para prevenir el cólera', *S*, 6 February 1991, p. 4; 'Chiclayo y playas en emergencia por temor a epidemias', *LI*(C), 6 February 1991, p. 1.

73. Municipalidad Provincial de Trujillo, 'Resolución de la Alcaldía'; and 'Piscinas estarán cerradas por 30 días en Trujillo', *S*, 15 and 18 February 1991, pp. 2, 3. The citation of '2 mil 500 kilos de pescado fueron ayer incinerados', in *S*, 7 February 1991, p. 3.
74. 'Dos toneladas de pescado descompuesto decomisan a ambulantes', *S*, 8 February 1991, p. 5.
75. 'Fiscal abrió investigación contra quienes riegan con aguas servidas', *LI*(C), 8 February 1991, p. 1.
76. Interview with Mallca Hernández.
77. 'Entrevista con César Bejarano, Director, Unidad de Tratamiento del Cólera del Hospital Cayetano Heredia, Piura', in *El Cólera, otro mal compañero de viaje*, CIPCA, Piura, 1991, pp. 8–9.
78. Diego Gonzales, 'El hospital bajo la furia del cólera', *Revista Médica Herediana*, **2**, 1992, pp. 54–6.
79. Javier Rios Davila, 'Impacto de la epidemia del colera y la huelga de salud en el servicio de emergencia, 1991', Medical thesis, Universidad Peruana Cayetano Heredia, 1993, p. 14.
80. Interview with Eyzaguirre Sotomayo.
81. Interview with Monge.
82. La Caleta received 7287 patients between 1 February and 2 March, 'Estadística oficial, cuadro pormenorizado del cólera', *DC*, 6 March 1991, p. 3.
83. Cited in 'La OPS en acción hoy en día: el caso del cólera', *Boletín de la Oficina Sanitaria Panamericana*, **71**, 113, 1992, pp. 374–5.
84. Interview with Rosado.
85. Interview with Jorge Ramal, 17 March 1996, former Director of the La Caleta Hospital.
86. Tocón and Acosta, *Con la vida*, p. 32; Marcela Chueca, Estrella Díaz and Paola Pérez, *Las mujeres y la alimentación popular ¿Una experiencia práctica de liberación femenina?* Celats, Lima, 1989.
87. Iturri, 'A Epidemia de cólera', p. 96.
88. Interview with Cuba. It was Cuba who phoned Fujimori to alert him of the epidemic.
89. Vidal was charged with 'health terrorism'. Mario Razzeto, 'Lima está a merced de toda plaga', *Oiga* (*O*), 18 February 1991, pp. 26–9. 'Cólera afecta al sector exportador', *RSD*, **14**, 608, 15–20 February 1991, p. 5.
90. Organización Panamericana de la Salud, *Riesgos de transmisión del cólera por los alimentos*, Organización Panamericana de la Salud, Washington, DC, 1991, p. 6.
91. 'Ecuador prohibe el ingreso de alimentos del Perú', and '86 muertos en primeros 10 días de cólera', *S*, 18 and 14 February 1991, pp. 3, 6–7. 'Control en Paraguay a viajeros llegados de Perú por el cólera', *LI*(C), 13 February 1991, p. 2.
92. Denise Koo, Héctor Traverso and Mario Libel, 'El cólera epidémico en América Latina: implicancias de las definiciones de casos usadas en la vigilancia sanitaria', *Revista Panamericana de Salud Pública*, **1**, 1997, pp. 85–92.
93. 'Perú perderá 300 millones de dólares al no poder exportar 250 mil toneladas de pescado', *S*, 18 February 1991, p. 3.
94. Margarita Petrera and Maibí Montoya, 'Impacto económico del cólera, Perú 1991', *Boletín Epidemiológico, Organización Panamericana de la Salud*, **13**, 2 September 1992, pp. 9–11. Petrera estimated that tourism fell in Peru by more than 90 per cent. J.D. Sneyder and P.A. Blake, 'Is Cholera a Problem for U.S. Travelers', *Journal of American Medical Association*, **247**, 1982, pp. 2268–9.

According to a later study the economic impact of cholera in 1991 was of US$176.9 million, including the costs per death. Suárez and Bradford, *Economic Impact*, p. 34.

95. 'Miles de pescadores sin trabajo en marcha comen pescados crudos para probar que no les pasa nada', *S*, 15 February 1991, p. 1.
96. 'Marcharon protestando pescadores artesanales y vendedores de pescado', *DC*, 16 February 1991, p. 1.
97. The statement was signed by the Subregional Office of the North-Eastern Region of the Marañón and the Fishermen's Syndicate. 'Un pronunciamiento frente a la sicosis del cólera', *LI*(C), 23 February 1991, p. 3.
98. 'Ministro defiende pescado', *DC*, 8 February 1991. From *ET*(P), 'Discrepancias en el gobierno', 'Ministerio de Pesquería hoy en Paita, Sechura y Caleta de Parachique' and 'No se registra víctimas por consumir alimentos peruanos', 2 and 3 March 1991, pp. 2, 5 and 7.
99. Carlos Reyna and Antonio Zapata, *Crónica sobre el cólera en el Perú*, Desco, Lima, 1991, p. 78.
100. 'Fujimori insiste', *RSD*, **14**, 609–10, 21 February–14 March 1991, p. 3.
101. 'Ministro de Salud, culpable del desastre', *O*, 25 February 1991, pp. 22–3.
102. 'Cuadrilátero político', *O*, 18 March 1991, p. 33.
103. 'Entrevista a Carlos Vidal, ex Ministro de Salud', *Medicamentos y Salud Popular*, **5**, 6 April 1991, p. 6.
104. 'La guerra del ceviche', p. 5.
105. The new Minister of Heath was Víctor Yamamoto. 'Punto final a la guerra del ceviche', *S*, 19 March 1991, p. 3; 'Rebrote colérico', *Caretas*, 4 March 1991, p. 43.
106. I gratefully acknowledge Dr Vidal for giving me a copy of his speech. Some physicians later admitted the recommendation 'do not eat raw fish' should have been changed to something more positive, like 'eat well-boiled fish'. Manuel Eyzaguirre, interview, Lima, 20 September 1996.
107. Ríos Dávila, 'Impacto de la epidemia'. The government declared the strike illegal.
108. '¡Drámatico llamado! No hay comisión ni apoyo para el cólera', *DC*, 21 February 1991, p. 1.
109. 'Ante asombro local: gobierno regional ayer destituyó a dos médicos', *DC*, 1 March 1991, p. 1; *RSD*, **14**, 612, 22–27 March 1991, p. 6.
110. Physical uncleanliness as a reflection of impurity and moral inferiority is an old topic in medicine. Owsei Temkin, 'An Historical Analysis of the Concept of Infection', in Owsei Temkin, *Studies in Intellectual History*, Johns Hopkins University Press, Baltimore, MD, 1953, pp. 123–47.
111. Marco Curatola, 'Mesías andinos, pestes, apocalípsis y el regreso de Cristo en el Perú privilegiado', *Historia y Cultura*, **21**, 1991–92, pp. 305–24.
112. Iturri, 'A Epidemia de cólera', p. 115.
113. Mary Fukumoto and Beth Yeager, *Percepciones de la población respecto del cólera*, Instituto de Investigación Nutricional, Lima, 1993, p. 14.
114. Ibid., p. 15.
115. 'También tenemos derecho, Deidamia Bautista, Chosica', in Jenny Menacho (comp.), *Cólera. La versión de los afectados*, PREDES, Chosica, 1991, p. 57. This book includes the testimonies of Juan Solórzano, Paulina Quispe and Deidamia Bautista.
116. On uncleanliness see Bruno Benavides, Roberto del Águila, Enrique Jacoby and Joaquín Novara, 'Conocimientos preventivos y de manejo de casos de cólera en

poblaciones de Lima y Piura luego de la epidemia', *Revista Peruana de Epistemiología*, **5**, 1, 1992, pp. 10–15.

117. The testimonies of Fany Gamboa Flores and Santos Esteban Cisneros, 27 and 33 years old, in 'Hospital Regional', *DC*, 6 February 1991, p. 4.
118. Iturri, 'A Epidemia de cólera', p. 135.
119. Roberto del Águila, Bruno Benavides, Enrique Jacoby and Joaquín Novara, 'Reconocimiento del cólera por personas sintomáticas después del brote epidémico en las UDES Sur y la subregión Luciano Castillo-Región Grau', *Revista Peruana de Epidemiología*, **5**, 1, 1992, p. 9.
120. 'También tenemos derecho', p. 57.
121. O. Mujica and Lourdes Gómez, 'Cólera en Perú: prevalencia de diarrea, exposición alimentaria y conocimientos, actitudes y prácticas, Ventanilla, Callao', *Revista Peruana de Epidemiología*, **4**, 2, 1991, pp. 51–61.
122. 'También tenemos derecho', p. 54.
123. 'Editorial: el castigo de la miseria, el cólera', *K*, 17 February 1991, p. 1.
124. 'Se confirmó que hay cólera pero también existe suciedad', *DC*, 6 February 1991, p. 1.
125. 'Triste es nuestra vida, Quispe', in Jenny Menacho (comp.), *Cólera. La versión de los afectados*, PREDES, Chosica, 1991, p. 42.
126. Carlos Carpio La Rosa, 'Pulso de la noticia', *DC*, 7 February 1991, p. 2.
127. According to a newspaper, the epidemic was due to the 'attitude of a people that does not love itself ... [and] lives amidst a permanent smell of filth and social injustice', '¿Dios nos ha abandonado?', p. 2.
128. The study was based on 53 families from shanty towns. R. Gilman, G.S. Marquis, G. Ventura, M. Campos, W. Spira and F. Díaz, 'Water Cost and Availability: Key Determinants of Family Higiene in a Peruvian Shantytown', *American Journal of Public Health*, **83**, 11, 1993, pp. 1554–8.
129. Interview with Alfredo Myres, 16 January 1996. He meant communities like Masitranka in Chota.
130. Carmela Gálvez and Dianera Regalado, 'Efectividad de 4 plantas de uso tradicional en el tratamiento de enfermedades parasitarias gastrointentinales de 1–5 años, Cajamarca, 1991', Licenciate thesis, Universidad Nacional de Cajamarca, 1991; Edin Alva (ed.), *El cólera, conversaciones campesinas sobre su presencia en Cajamarca*, Universidad de Cajamarca, Cajamarca, 1993. An infusion of guava leaves and lemon juice was also given in Iquitos. Fukumoto and Yeager, *Percepciones*, p. 16. For the variety of medicinal herbs promoted in Iquitos see Gobierno Regional de Loreto, *Diarrea, cuadernos divulgativos del tratamiento con plantas medicinales*, Agencia Española Cooperación Internacional, Iquitos, 1992; 'Dice alcalde de Pallasca: yerba milagrosa Paico cura el cólera', *DC*, 16 March 1991, p. 1; 'Herbolarios afirman que curan síntomas de cólera', *LI*(C), 19 February 1991, p. 6. Lemon juice is active against *Vibrio*, but the alkalinity of the water lowers it. Miguel Daquino and Sergio Teves, 'El limón como biocida natural para desinfectar las aguas de consumo', *Boletín de la Oficina Sanitaria Panamericana*, **4**, 117, 1994, pp. 289–95.
131. Just like other products, like garlic. *Luchemos contra el cólera*, Dirección Regional de Educación y Unidad Departamental de Salud, Piura, 1991, p. 1.
132. 'También tenemos derecho', p. 58.
133. 'Mi mamita ya no está, Juana Solórzano, Llacanora, Cajamarca', in Jenny Menacho (comp.), *Cólera. La versión de los afectados*, PREDES, Chosica, 1991, p. 19.
134. Iturri, 'A Epidemia de cólera', p. 98.

135. Haratani and Hernández, *Cholera in Peru*, p. xi.
136. 'La situación del cólera', pp. 13–16.
137. Iturri, 'A Epidemia de cólera', p. 151.
138. Fukumoto and Yeager, *Percepciones*, p. 18.
139. 'Intervención del Dr Guerra de Macedo, Director de la OPS', in Organización Panamericana de la Salud, *XXV Reunión del Consejo Directivo de la Organización Panamericana de la Salud, Actas Resumidas, Septiembre 23–27, 1991*, Organización Panamericana de la Salud, Washington, DC, 1991, p. 233.

CHAPTER SIX

Conclusions and Epilogue

Epidemics are dramatic crises which cause fear and despair, but also give both individuals and societies a chance to change and improve. The fear they cause is not just because they violently bring us close to a widespread disease and to death. Rather, they present what we sometimes fear the most in society and in other people: the authoritarian power that seems to be protecting us but which usually transgresses our individual rights, and the obligation to accept the fact that we live with people and groups we consider different, strange and even threatening to our physical well-being and our cultural identity. The despair caused by the epidemics studied in this book reflects the unstable living conditions of most of Peru's population, the deficiencies of the sanitation infrastructure and the lack of medical resources that often cannot help to prevent the avoidable deaths of a great number of children and adults. These epidemics also indicate that there was an epidemiological outline of twentieth-century Peru that stressed – real and perceived – geographical and social divisions.

In geographical terms epidemics seem to reinforce the separation between the people of the coast, the highlands and the tropical forest. The coast was considered a region where vector-produced, infectious diseases like yellow fever and malaria prevailed, and where its inhabitants acquired a certain degree of natural immunity. It was in this region that people migrating from the highlands got sick in large numbers. In the highlands, altitude and other ecological characteristics created a barrier against this type of disease. On the other hand, the absence of any health coverage and a way of life marked by poverty and the overcrowded living conditions of the peasants spread smallpox and typhus all over the highlands, and these were almost unknown on the coast. The tropical forest had similar characteristics, but these were more acute than those of the coast; here, the people from the highlands were also considered the group more at risk of contracting diseases the natives were more resistant to. These conditions heightened the fragmentation and divorce between the ethnic groups in the three classic regions into which Peru's geography is usually divided.

In social terms, epidemics separated the rich from the poor. The Chinese, the highlanders, the filthy: in several epidemics these groups seemed to be the dregs of society, those most infected and the ones to blame for the origin and spread of a disease. Some of the sanitary measures and the official and popular perceptions seemed to hold them responsible for any ailment and confirmed the gap between the elite and the poor, and between the pure and the dregs. These perceptions were also used to explain the limited results achieved. Actually, the lack of resources with which to carry out sanitation campaigns led to a confusion between protection, control and the desire for health on the one hand, and stigma, exclusion and segregation on the other. This confusion was heightened in a poor country like Peru, where diseases and stereotypes were used to justify the enormous social gaps, and the sometimes subtle ethnic differences.

The social and ethnic stigma associated with disease was not just the product of the medical conceptions of the time, but also a reflection of the cultural and political milieu in which the doctors lived. Furthermore, the suspicions held of the poor and the authoritarian nature of the campaigns reflected the overall authoritarian nature of Peruvian society and most governments throughout the twentieth century. In this way the vicious circle of underdevelopment and disease, of epidemics and poverty, and a frustrated modernization and unhealthiness, shows the permanence of social fragmentation and the weakness of the State in Peruvian society.

Peru's epidemiological chart gradually began to change with the relative control obtained in the campaigns against malaria which began after the 1940s, as the environmental barriers that hindered migration from the highlands to the coast and the tropical forest lost their significance. This led to the present situation: where some diseases (like yellow fever on the coast and smallpox in the highlands) have vanished; where the exchange of diseases between geographical regions has increased (for example, tuberculosis was almost exclusively a coastal disease prior to the 1940s, but then it expanded into the highlands); and where an epidemiological profile developed wherein old infectious diseases and chronic and degenerative ailments live side by side with similar intensity (although transmittable diseases continue to be the first cause of death in the country), thus making the transition to more civilized ways of living and dying difficult for Peru's population. Diseases no longer seem to be circumscribed to some regions, partly due to the massive migrations from the highlands to the coast, and partly because of this new epidemiological condition, and as a result the 'filthy' were responsible for the 1991 cholera outbreak – not any defined ethnic group, as in previous epidemics.

However, epidemics present excellent opportunities for institutional changes and improvements in living conditions and lifestyles. In a country with many pending tasks, epidemic diseases seem to have been the only occasion when public health caught the interest of the Peruvian government and international organizations. Sanitary emergencies were the stimuli for the adoption of measures which brought about an improvement, albeit a temporary one (including personal hygiene) and established new institutions, laws and processes that would mark the development of Peru's public health. This explains the formation of the first national health agency at the time of the bubonic plague, which gave work and prestige to health professionals, and established lasting contacts with US medicine and technical assistance, starting with the yellow fever epidemic which affected the north coast. Finally, at the time of the cholera epidemic the State and non-governmental organizations began to take a greater interest in environmental health conditions, and the hygiene of people improved.

However, with the hindsight of almost a century, the epidemics discussed in this book show the rise and fall of the importance that the Peruvian State accorded to public health. Just as the plague and the epidemic of yellow fever allowed the State to ascribe a greater significance to health, so the failure of the campaigns for the eradication of malaria and cholera helped make health lose some of its importance. The difference lay in part in the social and political context, for while the first was a moment of relative prosperity and stability, where the expansion of the State's powers were seen under a favourable light, the decline came during periods of a general crisis like the one in which cholera appeared, when the State began to be considered an anachronistic and bureaucratic institution that hampered economic development.

The difference can also be explained by the social actors involved in each epidemic event. In the early twentieth century, doctors and health workers managed to convince the politicians and the people that a nation-wide sanitary organization had to be developed; with the support of the Indian communities, Núñez Butrón managed in the 1930s to develop a creative public health system without significant support from the State. In contrast, with cholera there was a young, dedicated and innovative group in the Ministry of Health, but it was trapped in an administration for which part of the State's social policies had to be dismantled.

Bubonic plague, malaria, cholera and other infectious diseases still ravage Peru. At the close of the twentieth century bubonic plague has regained strength in the north, and so has malaria caused by *Plasmodium falciparum* on the coast and in the tropical forest.[1] Sylvan yellow fever furiously attacks Andean migrants moving to new frontiers areas in the Amazon. Tuberculosis poses a serious problem, as proved by the fact that Peru has one of the highest prevalences in all America, while the number of people infected with AIDS has increased since 1983 when the epidemic was first registered. Although the risk of acquiring transmittable diseases preventable by immunization has been reduced thanks to an improved programme of the Ministry of Health and other diseases like cholera have diminished (only 4518 cases were recorded in 1996), the causes that gave rise to the 655 548 cases accumulated between 1991 and 1996 have not been completely solved and the diarrhoeal diseases could regain strength due to the neglect of hygiene education and environmental sanitation. The major health indicators for Peru in 1996, like the rate of infant mortality (59 per 1000 born alive), the rate of mother mortality (261 per 100 000 children born alive), the number of physicians per 10 000 inhabitants (7.3), and the total expenditure in health as a percentage of the gross domestic product (3.1 per cent) suggest the enormous health challenges presented to Peruvians.[2] A reorganization of the sanitary services has been promoted from the Ministry but its impact on the epidemiological profile of the country is still to be seen. In brief, Peruvians still live under the shadow of epidemics, under the threat of an impending major sanitary crisis.

Something different can and needs to be done to break with the recurrence of disease and poverty. Both individuals and societies need a public health sector supported by the State, not just because this contributes to development but because it gives the citizens a feeling of security, hope, order and of equal opportunities. There is a possibility of giving new meanings to health that promote integration, citizenship, self-esteem and development. Public health can be developed in the face of adversity, as was shown by the case of Manuel Núñez Butrón, and by the behaviour of several doctors during epidemics, the cholera outbreak included.

To do so, the pattern of temporal responses as a function of emergencies needs to be apprehended and dropped. It means focusing efforts on preventive and essential primary health care, creatively using the few existing resources, carefully selecting appropriate and renewable technologies, establishing priorities according to local needs, effectively integrating domestic and traditional medicine into a national system of sanitary care, and promoting an active participation – with leadership roles – of various organizations, professionals and members of the community.

The redefinition of the participation of the State, non-governmental organizations and other institutions also entails becoming acquainted with the past experience of Peruvian public health as a vital matter for the establishment of a national sanitary culture. This kind of historical account should move beyond the institutional, celebratory and parochial historical model applied by the pioneers of the history of medicine in Peru. This study would like to suggest that the history of medicine cannot be just an account of hospitals, colleges, or what the physicians thought and did when looking after our health. What the patients or the people at large (many of whom had no access to western medicine) thought is just as important, if not more so. Such a study can improve our understanding of health and disease, and can reveal the relations of opposition and tolerance that took place between modern medicine and its domestic and traditional counterpart. This would likewise help us apprehend the problems that break up the dialogue between, and the productive co-existence of, different medical systems, and appreciate the good points and the weaknesses of popular conceptions of physical and mental well-being. This kind of history can help strengthen the elements of solidarity, integration and equality that will enable Peru to overcome the fragmentation and inequalities that criss-cross it, as well as help break the vicious circle of poverty and disease which regularly comes back to Peru as an epidemic.

Notes

1. See Organización Panamericana de la Salud y Ministerio de Salud, *Situación nacional de salud. Evaluación conjunta para la cooperación técnica*, Ministerio de Salud, Lima 1994, p. 10; Instituto Nacional de Estadística e Informática, *Perú: características de salud de la población*, Dirección Técnica de Demografía, Lima, 1997.
2. 'Situación del cólera en las Américas, 1996', *Boletín Epidemiológico, Organización Panamericana de la Salud*, 18, 1997, p. 7; 'Situación de salud en las Américas. Selección de indicadores básicos, 1996', *Boletín Epidemiológico, Organización Panamericana de la Salud*, 18, 1997, pp. 8–9.

Bibliography

Primary sources

Archives

Peru

Archivo de la Cámara de Comercio de Trujillo (ACCT)
Correspondencia Recibida, Years 1921–22.
Archivo Departamental de Ayacucho (ADA)
Serie Prefectura Ayacucho. Subserie Oficios Recibidos, Leg. 98, Years 1915–58.
Archivo Departamental de Cajamarca. (ADCa)
Serie Prefectura Cajamarca.
Subserie Libros copiadores de la Prefectura a los Ministerios, Leg. 655, Years 1904–11; Leg. 659, Years 1916–22.
Subserie Ministerio de Fomento, Leg. 220, Years 1909–12; Leg. 221, Years 1913–20; Leg. 222, Years 1921–29.
Archivo Departamental del Cuzco (ADCu)
Serie Prefectura Cuzco. Subserie Comunicaciones, Leg. 4, Years 1927–29; Leg. 7, Year 1932; Leg. 8, Year 1933; Leg.13, Year 1938; Leg. 19, Year 1948.
Serie Documentos de La Administración del Tesoro, Leg. 55, Year 1933.
Monografías de la Universidad San Antonio de Abad, Years 1944, 1946, 1947.
Archivo Departamental de Lambayeque (ADLa)
Concejo Provincial de Ferrañafe. Libro de Correspondencia, Years 1920–21.
Serie Prefectura Lambayeque. Subserie Ministerio de Fomento-Direccion de Salubridad, Year 1921.
Consejo Provincial de Chiclayo. Archivo Alcaldía. Libros Copiadores de Comunicaciones, Years 1904–06 and 1906–12.
Archivo Departamental de Piura (ADP)
Boletín de la Municipalidad de Piura, Years 1907–12.
Registro Oficial del Departamento de Piura, Year 1904.
Archivo Departamental de Puno, (ADPu)
Actuario Luis Rosado, Leg. 1261; Expedientes Judiciales 1935, Leg. 1261.
Varios actuarios, Leg. 224–36; Expedientes Judiciales 1940–50, Leg 224–36.
Archivo General de la Nación (AGN)
Fondo Archivo Agrario.

Serie Compañia Agrícola Cuzco Sociedad Anónima, CACSA, Subserie Correspondencia, Leg. 22 and 29.
Fondo Ministerio de Fomento.
Dirección de Salubridad Pública, Leg. 810–136, Year 1922.
Fondo Ministerio del Interior.
Prefectura Lima. Subprefectura Lima, Leg. 16, Year 1904.
Paquete 213, Year 1920.
Prefectura Cuzco, Paquete 331, Year 1933.
Archivo Histórico de la Biblioteca Municipal del Cuzco (AHBMC)
Leg. 94, Year 1932; Leg. 97, Year 1933.
Archivo Municipal de Paita (AMPa)
'Libro de Actas, Junta Incineradora, Tasadora y Pagadora, principiado el 5 de agosto de 1905'.
'Espanto sanitario', *La Igualdad*, 13 March 1906
Archivo Municipal de Piura (AMPi)
Boletín Municipal de Piura, Years 1907, 1909, 1912.
Expediente Municipal, Year 1911.
Biblioteca Nacional, Lima (BN)
Oficina de Investigaciones Bibliográficas y Fondos.
Papers of Manuel Núñez Butrón kept by Lourdes Núñez Guillén in Yanaura, Arequipa (PMNB-A).
Papers of Manuel Núñez Butrón kept by Rosa Jacinta Núñez in San Martín de Porres, Lima (PMNB-L).

Spain

Archivo General e Histórico de la Universidad de Barcelona (AGHUB)
Expediente Manuel Núñez Butrón.
Ficha 'Núñez Butrón, Manuel'.

USA

National Archives, Washington, DC (NA)
Record Group 90, United States Public Health Service, Foreign Governments, 'Peru' Box 37.
Records of State Relating to Internal Affairs of Peru, 1910–29. Political Affairs, Microfilm 4.
Rockefeller Archive Center, North Tarrytown, New York (RAC)
Rockefeller Foundation Archives (RFA)
R.G. 1.1, Series 331, Box 3.
R.G. 1.2, Series 331, Box 1.
R.G. 5, Series 1.1, Boxes 47, 56, 96; Series 1.2, Boxes 97, 117, 139; Series 2, Box 36; Series 3, Boxes 103, 104.

R.G. 12.1 William C. Gorgas, Diary, 1919.
Lewis Hackett collection.
Series 4, Box 19.

Interviews

Jaime Abad Coloma, Paita, 21 September 1989.
Eduardo Chuecas, Iquitos, 23 May 1996.
Victor Cuba, Lima, 8 January 1996.
Melchor Cutipa Coaquira, Juliaca, Puno, 1 July 1989.
Manuel Eyzaguirre, Lima, 20 September 1996.
Diomedes Mallca Hernandez, Cajamarca, 18 January 1996.
Zoila Mendoza-Walker, Cuzco, 21 June 1989.
Eduardo Monge, Lima, 18 September 1996.
Alfredo Myres, Cajamarca, 16 January 1996.
Rosa Jacinta Nuñez, Lima, 28, 30 August 1994.
Jorge Ramal, Chimbote, 17 March 1996.
Juan Rosado, Chimbote, 15 March 1996.
Mariano Velazquez García, Juliaca, 27 June 1989.

Secondary sources

Acosta, Manuel, 'Niveles Básicos de susceptibilidad del *Anopheles Pseudo-punctipennis* al DDT y al Dieldrin en la región occidental del Perú', *Revista de Medicina Experimental*, **12**, 1958, 99–106.

Acosta, Manuel, Napán, Marcelino and Villanueva, Carmen, 'Suceptibilidad y resistencia a los insecticidas de los vectores de malaria en el Perú', *Revista Médica Peruana*, **32**, 1963, 41–8.

Actividades de la Organización Mundial de la Salud, 1990–1991, Organización Mundial de la Salud, Geneva, 1992.

Agnoli, Juan B., *Memoria elevada a la Alcaldía por el Inspector de Higiene del Concejo Provincial de Lima, La Peste Bubónica en los años de 1903 y 1904*, Imp. Gil, Lima, 1905.

———, 'La peste en Lima, Informe que eleva a la Presidencia de la Junta Directiva de la Campaña contra la Peste Bubónica en la Provincia de Lima', *Boletín del Ministerio de Fomento*, **2**, 1906, 1–150.

Aguila, Roberto del, Benavides, Bruno, Jacoby, Enrique and Novara, Joaquín, 'Reconocimiento del cólera por personas sintomáticas después del brote epidémico en las UDES Sur y la sub-región Luciano Castillo-Región Grau', *Revista Peruana de Epidemiología*, **5**, 1, 1992, 5–9.

Aldana, Susana and Diez, Alejandro, *Balsillas, piajenos y algodón, procesos históricos en Piura y Tumbes*, CIPCA, Lima, 1994.

Almenara Irigoyen, Guillermo, *La racionalización de la salubridad pública*, Imp. Torres Aguirre, Lima, 1932.

Alva, Edin (ed.) *El cólera, conversaciones campesinas sobre su presencia en Cajamarca*, Universidad de Cajamarca, Cajamarca, 1993.

Alvan, José, 'Sanatorio militar para tuberculosos de la III y IV Divisiones', *Revista de Sanidad Militar*, **5**, 1932, 82–6.

Anderson, Christopcr, 'Cholera Epidemic Traced to Risk Miscalculation, Cancer Fear Lead to Halting of Chlorination', *Nature*, **354**, 28 November 1991, 255.

Arnold, David, *Colonizing the Body, State Medicine and Epidemic Disease in Nineteenth Century India*, University of California Press, Berkeley, CA, 1993.

Artola, Manuel, Arce, Julián, and Lavorería, Daniel E., *La peste bubónica: Informe Presentado a la Academia Nacional de Medicina*, Imp. Torres Aguirre, Lima, 1903.

Ayala, Juan L., *Insurgencia de los Yatiris, manifestaciones culturales del hombre andino*, Concytec, Lima, 1990.

Bachman, Carlos, *Departamento de Lambayeque, Monografía Histórico-Geográfica*, Imp. Torres Aguirre, Lima, 1921.

Barreda, Carlos, *La Industria de lanas en el Perú y en el departamento de Puno*, Imp. Torres Aguirre, Lima, 1929.

Barton, Alberto L., *La Lucha contra el paludismo*, Congreso Nacional de Medicina, Lima, 1927.

Barúa, Dhiman and Greenough, William B. (eds), *Cholera*, Plenum Medical, New York, 1992.

Basadre, Jorge, *Historia de la República del Perú*, 11 vols, Ed. Universitaria, Lima, 1969.

Bastien, Joseph, *Healers of the Andes: Kallawaya Herbalists and their Medicinal Plants*, University of Utah Press, Salt Lake City, UT, 1987.

Bastien, Joseph and Donahue, John, *Health in the Andes*, American Anthropological Association, Washington, DC, 1981.

Batchelor, R.A. and Wignall, S.F., 'Nontogenic 01 *Vibrio Cholerae* in Peru: A Report of Two Cases Associated with Diarrhea', *Diagnostic Microbiological Infectious Diseases*, **10**, 1988, 135.

Benavides, Bruno, 'Consumo de alimentos en comedores populares de Lima durante la epidemia de Cólera', *Revista Peruana de Epidemiología*, **4**, 2, 1991, 102–8.

Benavides, Bruno, Del Aguila, Roberto, Jacoby, Enrique and Novara, Joaquín, 'Conocimientos preventivos y de manejo de casos de cólera en poblaciones de Lima y Piura luego de la epidemia', *Revista Peruana de Epidemiología*, **5**, 1, 1992, 10–15.

Bendiner, E., 'Noguchi: Many Triumphs and a Brilliant Failure', *Hospital Practice*, **19**, 1984, 222–7.

Bertram, Geoff, 'Modernización y cambio en la industria lanera en el sur del Perú, 1919–1930, un caso frustrado de desarrollo', *Apuntes*, **3**, 1977, 3–22.

Besser, Richard E., Moscoso, Betsy, Cabanillas, Oswaldo, Gonzáles, Liduvira, Minaya, Percy, Ridríguez, Marcela, Saldaña, Wilton, Seminario, José Luis, Highsmith, Anita K. and Tauxe, Robert V., 'Prevención de la transmisión del cólera: evaluación rápida de la calidad del agua municipal en Trujillo, Perú', *Boletín de la Oficina Sanitaria Panamericana*, **119**, 3, 1995, 189–94.

Bethel, Leslie (ed.), *Latin America: Economy and Society, 1870–1930*, Cambridge University Press, Cambridge, 1989.

Biffi, Ugo, *Saneamiento de Lima*, Imp. Gil, Lima, 1903.

Blake, Paul A., 'Epidemiology of Cholera in the Americas', *Gastroenterology Clinics of North America*, **22**, 3 1993, 639–60.

Bourricaud, Francois, *Cambios en Puno: Estudios de Sociología andina*, Instituto Indigenista Interamericano, México, 1967.

Brown, C.V., and Nossal, G.J., 'Malaria, Yesterday, Today, and Tomorrow', *Perspectives in Biology and Medicine*, **20**, 1, 1986, 65–76.

Brown, E. Richard, 'Public Health and Imperialism: Early Rockefeller Programs at Home and Abroad', *American Journal of Public Health*, **66**, 9, 1976, 897–903.

Burga, Manuel and Flores Galindo, Alberto, *Apogeo y Crisis de la República Aristocrática*, Ed. Rickchay Perú, Lima, 1980.

Butler, Thomas, *Plague and Other Yersinia Infections*, Plenum Medical, New York, 1983.

Cámara de Diputados, *Diario de debates, Congreso Ordinario de 1904*, El Comercio, Lima, 1904.

Carter, Henry R., *Yellow Fever: An Epidemiological and Historical Study of its Place of Origin*, Williams and Wilkins, Baltimore, MD, 1931.

Carvallo, Constantino, *Memoria del Ministro de Salud Pública y Asistencia Social, 1941–1945*, Imp. Torres Aguirre, Lima, 1945.

Castro, Lucio D., 'El Chujchu, folklore andino', *Perú Indígena*, **4**, 1953, 100–105.

Castro Pozo, Hildebrando, *Nuestra Comunidad Indígena*, Ed. El Lucero, Lima, 1924.

Censo Nacional de Población y Ocupación de 1940, 1, Ministerio de Hacienda, Lima, 1944.

Chávez, Nazario, *Cajamarca*, 2 vols, Talleres Leoncio Prado, Lima, 1957.

Chiriboga, Jorge, *La Malaria en los Valles de 'La Convención', Andes Orientales del Sur del Perú*, Librería Miranda, Lima, 1947.

Chiriboga, Jorge and Donayre, Rafael, *Epidemiología en los Andes y el problema de las migraciones humanas*, Dirección de Salubridad Pública, Lima, 1948.

'Cholera in the Americas', *Weekly Epidemiological Record, World Health Organization*, **67**, 1992, 33.

'Cholera-Peru, 1991', *Journal of the American Medical Association*, **10**, 265, 1991, 1232.

'Cholera-Peru, 1991', *Morbidity and Mortality Weekly Report, Centers for Disease Control*, **40**, 1991, 108.

Chueca, Marcela, Diaz, Estrella and Perez, Paola, *Las mujeres y la alimentación popular ¿Una experiencia práctica de liberación femenina?* Celats, Lima, 1989.

Cieza, Javier, 'Esquema para el manejo de pacientes deshidratados por cólera', *Revista Médica Herediana*, **2**, 1991, 68–9.

Cipolla, Carlos M., *Fighting the Plague in Seventeenth-Century Italy*, University of Wisconsin Press, Madison, WI, 1981.

Cisneros, Carlos B., 'Monografía de Lima', *Boletín de la Sociedad Geográfica de Lima*, **26**, 1910, 179.

Clark, Paul F., 'Hideyo Noguchi 1876–1928', *Bulletin of the History of Medicine*, **33**, 1959, 1–20.

Coleman, William, *Yellow Fever in the North: The Methods of Early Epidemiology*, University of Wisconsin Press, Madison, WI, 1987.

'El Cólera en las Américas, Actualización', *Boletín Epidemiológico, Organización Panamericana de la Salud*, **12**, 2, 1991, 1–2.

Comisión Interinstitucional de Estadísticas del Medio Ambiente, *Perú, Estadísticas del medio ambiente*, Instituto Nacional de Estadística e Informática, Lima, 1993.

Cook, Noble David, *Demographic Collapse: Indian Peru, 1520–1620*, Cambridge University Press, Cambridge, 1981.

Cooper, Donald B., *Epidemic Disease in Mexico City, 1761–1813: An Administrative, Social and Medical Study*, University of Texas Press, Austin, TX, 1965.

Corporación Departamental de Desarrollo de Cajamarca, *Problemáticas y perspectivas de desarrollo del departamento de Cajamarca 1983–1985*, CDDC, Lima, 1983.

Corradetti, Augusto, *Bases experimentales para la eliminación de la malaria en la costa del Perú*, Dirección de Salubridad Pública, Lima, 1947.

Cotler, Julio, *Clases, Estado y Nación en el Perú*, Instituto de Estudios Peruanos, Lima, 1978.

Craig, Wesley W., *From Hacienda to Community: An Analysis of Solidarity and Social Change in Peru*, Cornell University American Studies Program, Ithaca, NY, 1967.

'Creación del Ministerio de Salud Pública, Trabajo y Previsión Social, Ley 8124', *Boletín de la Dirección de Salubridad Pública*, 1935, 3–4, El Universal, Lima, 1935.

Crosby, Alfred W., *The Columbian Exchange: Biological and Cultural Consequences of 1492*, Greenwood Press, Westport, CT, 1972.

Cuadros, F., *El Arriendo y la reforma agraria en el Cuzco*, H.G. Rosas, Cuzco, 1949.

Cueto, Marcos, *Excelencia científica en la periferia, actividades científicas e investigación biomédica en el Perú, 1890–1950*, Tarea, Lima, 1989.

———, 'Andean Biology in Peru: Scientific Styles in the Periphery', *Isis*, **80**, 1989, 640–58.

———, 'Indigenismo and Rural Medicine in Peru: The Indian Sanitary Brigade and Manuel Nuñez Butrón', *Bulletin of the History of Medicine*, **65**, 1991, 22–41.

——— (ed.), *Missionaries of Science: The Rockefeller Foundation and Latin America*, Indiana University Press, Bloomington, IN, 1994.

———, (ed.), *Salud, Cultura y Sociedad en América Latina: Nuevas Perspectivas Históricas*, Instituto de Estudios Peruanos/Organización Panamericana de la Salud, Lima, 1996.

Cunningham, Andrew, 'Transforming Plague: The Laboratory and the Identity of Infectious Disease', in Andrew Cunningham and Perry Williams (eds), *The Laboratory Revolution in Medicine*, 209–44, Cambridge University Press, Cambridge, 1992.

Curátola, Marco, 'Mesías andinos, pestes, apocalípsis y el regreso de Cristo en el Perú privilegiado', *Historia y Cultura*, **21**, 1991–92, 305–24.

Dáquino, Miguel and Teves Sergio, A., 'El limón como biocida natural para desinfectar las aguas de consumo', *Boletín de la Oficina Sanitaria Panamericana*, **4**, 117, 1994, 289–95.

Delaporte, Francois, *Disease and Civilization, the Cholera in Paris, 1832*, Massachusetts Institute of Technology, Cambridge, MA, 1986.

Delgado Bedoya, Gabriel, 'Doctrina y acción *rijchary* de Manuel Núñez Butrón', *Medicina Social*, **10**, 1953, 8–10.

Dew, Edward, *Politics in the Altiplano: The Dynamics of Change in Rural Peru*, University of Texas Press, Austin, TX, 1969.

Dobyns, Henry F., 'An Outline of Andean Epidemic History to 1720', *Bulletin of the History of Medicine*, **37**, 1963, 493–515.

Dourejanni, Marc J. (ed.), *Gran Geografía del Perú*, 5 vols, Manfer-Juan Mejía Baca, Lima, 1986.

Durey, Michael, *The Return of the Plague, British Society and the Cholera, 1831–1832*, Gill and Macmillan Humanities Press, Dublin, 1979.

Downs, W.G., 'History of Epidemiological Aspects of Yellow Fever', *Yale Journal of Biology and Medicine*, **55**, 1982, 179–85.

'Encuesta para conocer la epidemiología nacional, Departamento de Cajamarca', *Boletín de la Dirección de Salubridad Pública*, 1919, 210–12, La Opinión Nacional, Lima, 1919.

Las Enfermedades transmisibles en el Perú, 1956, Ministerio de Salud Pública y Asistencia Social y Servicio Cooperativo Interamericano de Salud Pública, Lima, June 1957.

'Entrevista a Carlos Vidal, ex Ministro de Salud', *Medicamentos y Salud Popular*, **5**, 6 April, 1991, 6.

'Epidemia del Cólera en el Perú, pautas para su control', *Boletín de la Oficina Sanitaria Panamericana*, **110**, 4, 1991, 277–97.

Eskey, C.R., 'Epidemiological Study of Plague in Peru', *Public Health Reports*, **47**, 18 November 1932, 2191–207.

Estrella Ruiz, J.A., 'La sanidad peruana en cincuenta años: apuntes para su historia', *Salud y Bienestar Social*, **6**, 1953, 92.

'Evaluación de las vacunas contra el cólera', *Boletín Epidemiologico, Organización Panamericana de la Salud*, **12**, 2, 1991, 11–12.

Evans, Richard J., *Death in Hamburg, Society and Politics in the Cholera Years, 1830–1910*, Penguin Books, London, 1987.

Eyzaguirre, Rómulo, 'Enfermedades evitables', *La Crónica Médica*, **20**, 1903, 1–5.

———, *La mortalidad de los lactantes de Lima, sus causas y sus remedios*, Imp. San Pedro, Lima, 1908.

Fee, Elizabeth and Fox, Daniel M. (eds), *AIDS: The Burdens of History*, University of California Press, Berkeley, CA, 1990.

Fenner, F., Henderson, D.A., Arita, I., Jezëk, Z. and Ladnyi, I.D., *Smallpox and its Eradication*, World Health Organization, Geneva, 1988.

Fernández, Faustuo, 'Endemo-epidemiología de la malaria en el Perú', *Salud y Bienestar Social*, **1**, 1953, 35–6.

'La fiebre amarilla, medios de evitarla', *Boletín de la Dirección de Salubridad Pública*, 1919, 37–41, La Opinión Nacional, Lima, 1919.

Fioravanti, Eduardo, *Latifundio y sindicalismo agrario en el Perú*, Instituto de Estudios Peruanos, Lima, 1976.

'El Fondo Nacional de Salud y Bienestar Social', *Salud y Bienestar Social*, **2**, 1953, 16.

Franco Agudelo, Saúl, 'El Saldo Rojo de los insecticidas en América Latina, a propósito de su utilización contra la malaria', *Revista Centro Americana de Ciencias de la Salud*, **20**, 1978, 35–54.

———, 'The Rockefeller Foundation's Antimalarial Program in Latin America: Donating or Dominating?', *International Journal of Health Services*, **13**, 1, 1983, 51–7.

———, *El Paludismo en América Latina*, University of Guadalajara, Guadalajara, 1990.

Frisancho Pineda, David, *Jatun Rijchari: Dr. Manuel Nuñez Butrón, precursor de la sanidad rural en el Perú*, Ed. Los Andes, Puno, 1958.

———, *Medicina indígena y popular*, Ed. Los Andes, Puno, 1988.

Fukumoto, Mary and Yeager, Beth, *Percepciones de la población respecto del cólera*, Instituto de Investigación Nutricional, Lima, February 1993.

Gamio, Enrique, 'La vivienda del indio como problema nacional', *Perú Indígena*, **2**, 1952, 17–39.

Garret, Laurie, *The Coming Plague, Newly Emerging Diseases in a World Out of Balance*, Penguin Books, New York, 1995.

Gastañaga, María del Carmen, 'Agua y saneamiento básico, Perú, 1991', *Revista Peruana de Epidemiologia*, **4**, 2, 1991, 70–85.

Gerbi, Antonello, *El Perú en marcha*, Banco Italiano de Cultura, Lima, 1941.

Gilman, R., Barúa, Raul León and Ramírez-Ramos, A., 'Significado de la infección por *Campylobacter pylori* en el Perú', *Acta Herediana*, **9**, 1988, 12–16.

Gilman, R., Marquis, G.S., Ventura, G., Campos, M., Spira, W. and Diaz, F., 'Water Cost and Availability: Key Determinants of Family Hygiene in a Peruvian Shantytown', *American Journal of Public Health*, **83**, 11, 1993, 1554–8.

Glass, R.I., Holmgren, J., Haley, C.E., Khan, M.R. Svennerholm, A.M., Stoll, B.J., Belayet Hossain, K.M., Black, R.E., Yunus, M. and Barua, D., 'Predisposition for Cholera of Individuals with O Blood Group: Possible Evolutionary Significance', *American Journal of Epidemiology*, **232**, 1985, 791–6.

Glass, R.I., Liberl, M. and Brandling-Bennet, A.D., 'Epidemic Cholera in the Americas', *Science*, **256**, 12 June 1992, 1524–5.

Gobierno Regional de Loreto, *Diarrea, cuadernos divulgativos del tratamiento con plantas medicinales*, Agencia Española de Cooperación Internacional, Iquitos, 1992.

Gomez, Luis M., 'Sobre la peste bubónica en Sullana, Febrero 8, 1919', *Boletín de la Dirección de Salubridad Pública*, 1919, 128–33, La Opinión Nacional, Lima, 1919.

Gomez Cumpa, José and Bazán, Inés, *Capitalismo y región en Lambayeque, 1879–1930*, Naylamp, Chiclayo, 1981.

Gonzales, Diego, 'El hospital bajo la furia del cólera', *Revista Médica Herediana*, **2**, 1992, 54–6.

Gonzalez, Michael J., *Plantation Agriculture and Social Control in Northern Peru, 1875–1933*, University of Texas Press, Austin, TX, 1985.

González Prada, Manuel, *Horas de lucha*, Ed. Universo, Lima, 1972.

Gotuzzo, Eduardo, 'El cólera en el Perú', *Revista Médica Herediana*, **2**, 3, 1991, 105–7.

'La Gran Cruzada Sanitaria', *Medicina Social*, **9**, 1952, 10–13.

Graña, Francisco, *La población del Perú a través de la historia*, Imp. Torres Aguirre, Lima, 1940.

Guillén, Eduardo, 'Algunas experiencias del Servicio Nacional de Erradicación de la Malaria con las tribus de la selva peruana', *Boletín de la Oficina Sanitaria Panamericana*, **52**, 1962, 143–5.

Hackett, Lewis W., 'La Medición del bazo en la malaria', *Revista de Medicina Experimental*,**11**,1943, 305–19.

———, 'The Malaria of the Andean Region of South America', *Revista del Instituto de Salubridad y Enfermedades Tropicales (Mexico)*, **6**, 4, 1945, 239–52.

Handelman, Howard, *Struggle in the Andes: Peasant Political Mobilization in Peru*, University of Texas Press, Austin, TX, 1975.

Hanson, Henry, 'The Sanitation of Paita', *West Coast Leader*, **9**, 436, 1920, 2.

———, *A Study of Sanitary Conditions in Peru with Special Reference to the Incidence of Malaria*, Panama Canal Press, Mount Hope, 1921.

———, *The Pied Piper of Peru: Dr. Henry Hanson's Fight against 'Yellow Jack' and Bubonic Plague in South America, 1919–1922*, Convention Press, Jacksonville, FL, 1961.

Haratani, Joseph and Hernandez, Donald, *Cholera in Peru: A Rapid Assessment of the Country's Water and Sanitation Infrastructure*, USAID Mission to Peru, Washington, DC, 1991.

Harrison, G., *Mosquitoes, Malaria and Man: A History of the Hostilities since 1880*, E.P. Dalton, New York, 1978.

Harrison, Mark, *Public Health in British India, Anglo-Indian Preventive Medicine, 1859–1914*, Cambridge University Press, Cambridge, 1994.

Hazen, Dan C., 'Meanings of Literacy in the Third World: The Concepts and Consequences of the *Rijchary* Reform Movement in Highland Peru', *Journal of Library History*, **16**, 1981, 404–15.

Hobsbawm, Eric, 'A Case of Neofeudalism: La Convención, Peru', *Journal of Latin American Studies*, **1**, 1969, 35–48.

Los Hombres de Kishuar, la medicina en la tradición Cajamarquina, Aspaderuc-PEC, Cajamarca, 1991.

Hopkins, Donald, *Princes and Peasants, Smallpox in History*, University of Chicago Press, Chicago, 1983.

Hoyos, César, Romero, Jorge and Monteverde, Luis, 'Rebrote epidémico del cólera en Lima', *Revista de Gastroenterología Peruana*, **12**, 1992, 26.

Informe Anual del Servicio Cooperativo Interamericano de Salud Pública, Ministerio de Salud Pública y Asistencia Social, Lima, 1957.

Instituto Nacional de Estadística e Informática, *Región Loreto, compendio estadístico, 1991–1992*, Dirección Nacional de Estadísticas Regionales, Lima, 1992.

Instituto Nacional de Estadística e Informática, *Perú: caracteristicas de salud de la población*, Dirección Técnica de Demografía, Lima, 1997.

International Health Board, *The Use of Fish for Mosquito Control*, Rockefeller Foundation, New York, 1924.

Jacobsen, Nils, *Mirages of Transition, the Peruvian Altiplano, 1780–1930*, University of California Press, Berkeley, CA, 1993.

Jiménez, Vicente A., *Apuntes Geográficos del Departamento de Puno*, Tipografía Fournier, Puno, 1924.

Kapsoli, Wilfredo (ed.), *Los Movimientos campesinos en el Perú, 1879–1965*, Delva Editores, Lima, 1977.

———, 'Movimientos sociales en Cayaltí, 1915–1919', *Allpanchis*, **11**, 1978, 103–22.

Kay, B.A. and Sack, R.B., '*Vibrio cholerae* non-01 Isolated from Five People with Diarrhoea in Lima', *Lancet*, **28**, 1, 1984, 218.

Kiple, Kenneth F. (ed.), *Cambridge World History of Human Disease*, Cambridge University Press, Cambridge, 1993.

Klaiber, Jeffrey, *La Iglesia en el Perú*, Pontificia Universidad Católica del Perú, Lima, 1988.

Klaren, Peter F., *Modernization, dislocation and Aprismo: Origins of the peruvian Aprista party, 1870–1932*, University of Texas Press, Austin, TX, 1973.

Klinge, Gerardo, *Arroz y malaria*, Sociedad Nacional Agraria, Lima, 1932.

———, *La agricultura de la costa y la situación alimentaria*, Sociedad Nacional Agraria, Lima, 1944.

Koo, Denise, Travers, Héctor and Libel, Mario, 'El cólera epidémico en América Latina: implicancias de la definiciones de casos usadas en la vigilancia sanitaria', *Revista Panamericana de Salud Pública*, **1**, 1997, 85–92.

Kristal, Efraín, *Una Visión Urbana de los Andes: Génesis y Desarrollo del Indigenismo en el Perú, 1848–1930*, Instituto de Apoyo Agrario, Lima, 1991.

Kuczynski Godard, Maxime, *Una Inspección preliminar de las zonas del Tifus andino*, Ed. La Reforma Médica, Lima, 1940.

———, *El Departamento de Amazonas, algunas observaciones médico sociales*, Imp. Americana, Lima, 1940.

———, *La Vida en la Amazonia Peruana, observaciones de un médico*, Librería Internacional del Perú, Lima, 1944.

———, *Estudios Médicos de la región sur del Perú*, Ministerio de Salud Pública y Asistencia Social, Lima, 1945.

———, *A Propósito del saneamiento de los valles Yungas del Cuzco (La Convención, Lares y Ocobamba)*, Ministerio de Salud Pública y Asistencia Social, Lima, 1946.

Kuon Cabello, Guillermo, 'Tifus exantemático en Tarata, Tacna', *La Crónica Médica*, **66**, 1949, 141–5.

'Labor del Servicio Nacional Antimalárico', *Boletín de la Dirección de Salubridad Pública*, 1944, 145–57, Imp. Miranda, Lima, 1945.

Lastres, Juan B, *Historia de la Medicina Peruana*, 3 vols, Universidad de San Marcos, Lima, 1951.

———, *La Salud Pública y la prevención de la viruela en el Perú*, Imp. del Ministerio de Hacienda y Comercio, Lima, 1957.

Luchemos contra el cólera, Dirección Regional de Educación y Unidad Departamental de Salud, Piura, 1991.

Litsios, Sócrates, 'Lucha antipalúdica y servicios epidemiológicos: ¿Hacia una nueva orientación?', *Foro Mundial de la Salud*, **14**, 1993, 45–54.

León García, Enrique, *Las razas en Lima*, Sanmartí y Cía, Lima, 1909.

Long, John D., 'Cooperative Campaign for the Eradication of Plague in Peru', *Public Health Report*, **37**, 11 September 1931, 2164.

Lopez Albujar, Enrique, *Los caballeros del delito. Estudio criminológico del bandolerismo en algunos departamentos del Perú*, Impresiones y Publicidad, Lima, 1936.

Lorente, Sebastián, 'La Obra médico social del gobierno del Señor Leguía', *Boletín de la Dirección de Salubridad Pública*, 1927, 133–8, Minerva, Lima, 1928.

Lorente, Sebastián and Flores, Raúl, *Estudios sobre Geografía Médica y Patología del Perú*, Imp. Americana, Lima, 1925.

Loyola, Luis Antonio, *La epidemia de cólera en el Perú y relación con los problemas de salud ambiental*, Organización Panamericana de la Salud, Lima, 1991.

Macchiavello, Atilio, 'Estudios sobre peste selvática en América del Sur, II', *Boletín de la Oficina Sanitaria Panamericana*, **43**, 1957, 226.

———, 'Estudios sobre la peste selvática en América del Sur, III', *Boletín de la Oficina Sanitaria Panamericana*, **44**, 1958, 484–512.

MacLeod, Roy and Lewis, Milton (eds), *Disease, Medicine and Empire, Perspectives on Western Medicine and the Experience of European Expansion*, Routledge, London, 1988.

Madueño, Jorge, 'La malaria causada por las obras de irrigación', *Boletín de la Escuela Nacional de Ingenieros*, **18**, 1945, 7–16.

———, 'El ingeniero y su intervención en el control de la malaria en el país', *Boletín de la Escuela Nacional de Ingenieros*, **22**, 1949, 51–72.

Marroquín, José, 'La medicina indígena puneña', *Anales de la Sociedad Peruana de Historia de la Medicina*, **2**, 1940, 42–57.

———, 'El problema sanitario indígena en Puno', *Medicina Social*, **2**, 1944, 6.

———, *La Sanidad rural indígena en el Departamento de Puno*, Tipografía Fournier, Puno, 1945.

———, 'Plan de acción sanitaria contra el Tifus exantemático en el Perú', *La Crónica Médica*, **66**, 1949, 72–4.

———, 'Estudio sanitario de un area rural en el altiplano puneño', *Salud y Bienestar Social*, **3**, 1954, 27.

Martínez, Ezequiel A., *La decadencia de la Facultad de Ciencias Médicas durante la administración del Dr. Carlos Villarán*, Imp. Samamé, Lima, 1937.

Mata, Leonardo, *El cólera, historia, prevención y control*, University of Costa Rica, San José, 1992.

Mcllellan, Scott, 'La muerte como modo de vida: el cólera mata pero la epidemia en el Perú también ha salvado vidas', *CERES, Revista de la FAO*, **24**, 137, 1992, 39–43.

McNeill, William H., *Plagues and Peoples*, Doubleday, New York, 1976.

Menacho, Jenny (comp.), *Cólera. La versión de los Afectados*, PREDES, Chosica, 1991.

Mendiburu, Armando and Foronda, María Elena, *Sondeo epidemiológico de los efectos de la contaminación industrial en Chimbote*, Natura, Chimbote, 1991.

Menendez Rua, Angel, *Paso a la civilización, obra histórica en la que se estudia el aspecto religioso y su desenvolvimiento en la provincia de La Convención*, Sanmartí, Lima, 1948.

Miller, Rory, 'The Coastal Elite and Peruvian Politics, 1895–1919', *Journal of Latin American Studies*, **82**, 1982, 97–120.

———, 'The Wool Trade of Southern Peru, 1850–1915', *Ibero-Amerikanisches Archiv*, **8**, 1982, 297–312.

Ministerio de Fomento, *Anales de las obras públicas del Perú*, Ministerio de Fomento, Lima, 1920.

Ministerio de Hacienda y Comercio, *Estado de la Instrucción en el Perú según el censo nacional de 1940*, Imp. Torres Aguirre, Lima, 1942.

Ministerio de Salud, *Legislación sanitaria, laboral, alimentaria, leyes, decretos, reglamentos y resoluciones*, Talleres de la Comandancia General de Aeronáutica, Lima, 1941.

———, *Legislación sanitaria peruana sobre alimentos, enfermedades transmisibles, estupefacientes y medicamentos*, Ministerio de Salud, Lima, 1974.

———, *Hacia un Sistema Nacional Regionalizado e Integrado de Salud (objetivos, políticas, metas)*, Ministerio de Salud, Lima, 1990.

Miró Quesada, Oscar, *Elementos de geografía científica del Perú*, El Comercio, Lima, 1919.

Molina, Gustavo E., *Salud ocupacional y epidemiología ambiental en la producción manufacturera de acero en Chimbote*, Centro Panamericano de Ecología Humana y Salud, Lima, 1982.

Moll, Arístides and Baughman O'Leary, Shirley, 'Plague in the Americas, Perú', *Boletín de la Oficina Sanitaria Panamericana*, **20**, 1941, 700.

Mujica, Oscar and Gómez, Lourdes, 'Cólera en Perú: Prevalencia de diarrea, exposición alimentaria y conocimientos, actitudes y prácticas, Ventanilla, Callao', *Revista Peruana de Epidemiología*, **4**, 2, 1991, 51–61.

Mujica, Oscar, Quick, Robert E., Palacios, Ana Mariá, Beingolea, Luis, Vargas, Rodolfo, Moreno, Dafne and Seminario, Luis, 'Cólera en la selva peruana: factores de riesgo y protección', *Revista Peruana de Epidemiología*, **4**, 2, 1991, 62–9.

Nájera, José A., 'El paludismo y las actividades de la Organización Mundial de la Salud', *Boletín de la Oficina Sanitaria Panamericana*, **111**, 1991, 131–51.

———, 'The Control of Tropical Diseases and Socioeconomic Development', *Parassitologia*, **36**, 1994, 17–33.

Núñez Butrón, Manuel, '¿Qué es el Rijcharismo?', *Medicina Social*, **2**, 1944, 9–10.

Olaechea, Abel S., 'Antecedentes de la ley de profilaxia del paludismo', *Boletín de Salubridad Pública*, 1917, 17, La Opinión Nacional, Lima, 1917.

———, 'Breve estudio de la situación higiénica y asistencia del Perú en el período comprendido desde fines del siglo XVIII y la época presente', *Revista Médica Peruana*, **5**, 1933, 612–39.

'La Organización de los servicios sanitarios en el Perú', *Boletín de la Dirección de Salubridad Pública*, 1927, 3–48, Imp. Americana, Lima, 1927.

Organización Panamericana de la Salud, *Riesgos de transmisión del cólera por los alimentos*, Organización Panamericana de la Salud, Washington, DC, 1991.

Organización Panamericana de la Salud, *XXV Reunión del Consejo Directivo de la Organización Panamericana de la Salud, Actas Resumidas, Septiembre 23–27, 1991*, Organización Panamericana de la Salud, Washington, DC, 1991.

———, *Las condiciones de salud en las Américas, 1994*, Organización Panamericana de la Salud, Publicación Científica 459, Washington, DC, 1994.

Organización Panamericana de la Salud y Ministerio de Salud, *Situación nacional de salud. Evaluación conjunta para la cooperación técnica*, Ministerio de Salud, Lima, 1994.

'Organización Sanitaria Nacional', *Boletín de la Dirección de Salubridad Pública*, 1935, 5–7, Dirección de Salubridad Pública, Lima, 1935.

'La OPS en acción hoy en día: el caso del cólera', *Boletín de la Oficina Sanitaria Panamericana*, **71**, 113, 1992, 374–5.

'El paludismo en La Convención y Lares, opinión de la Academia Nacional de Medicina', *La Crónica Médica*, **50**, 1933, 343–5.

Parks, Lois F. and Nuermberger, Gustave A., 'The Sanitation of Guayaquil', *Hispanic American Historical Review*, **23**, 1943, 197–221.

Paz Soldán, Carlos Enrique, *La pandemia malárica en los valles cálidos del Cuzco*, Instituto de Medicina Social, Lima, 1903.

———, *La Región Cuzco-Puno, estudio médico militar*, Servicio Geográfico del Ejército, Lima, 1933.

———, 'El saneamiento rural de la costa peruana', *La Reforma Médica*, **5**, 1919, 75–86.

———, *La sanidad pública en el Perú*, Imp. Torres Aguirre, Lima, 1920.

———, 'El Dominio de la Selva por la medicina social', *Boletín de la Sociedad Geográfica de Lima*, **37**, 1921, 54–6.

———, *Una Cruzada patriótica por la salud de los trabajadores del campo, la*

demostración de asistencia y saneamiento rural del valle de Carabayllo, Ed. Rímac, Lima, 1933.

———, *La Peste Verde*, Instituto de Medicina Social, Lima, 1934.

———, *El Malarigenismo del valle de Cañete*, La Reforma Médica, Lima, 1936.

———, *La Selva Peruana, sus pobladores y su colonización en seguridad sanitaria*, Imp. Lux, Lima, 1939.

Paz Soldán, Carlos Enrique and Kuczynski Godard, Maxime, *La Colonia del Perené y sus problemas médico sociales*, La Reforma Médica, Lima, 1939.

Pesce, Luis, *Indigenismo e inmigrantes en el Perú*, Imp. de la Opinión Nacional, Lima, 1906.

Petrera, Margarita and Montoya, Maibi, 'Impacto económico del cólera, Perú 1991', *Boletín Epidemiológico, Organización Panamericana de la Salud*, **13**, 2 September 1992, 9–11.

Pollitzer, R., *Plague*, World Health Organization, Geneva, 1954.

———, *Cholera*, World Health Organization, Geneva, 1959.

Polo, José Toribio, *Apuntes sobre las epidemias en el Perú*, Federico Barrionuevo, Lima, 1913.

'Por qué no salen los médicos a provincias', *La Acción Médica*, **6**, 4 February 1928, 12.

Portella, Juan, *Datos demográficos de la ciudad de Lima en 1904*, Imp. Lucero, Lima, 1905.

Portugal, José, *José Antonio Encinas: el maestro de los maestros peruanos*, Concytec, Lima, 1986.

Portugal, Julio E., 'La sanidad en el Perú', *Boletín de la Dirección de Salubridad Pública*, 1947, 8–17, Minerva, Lima, 1947.

'El Problema de las Basuras de Lima', *La Crónica Médica*, **80**, 1925, 19–20.

Programa de las Naciones Unidas para el Desarrollo, *Informe Anual de la Cooperación para el Desarrollo, Peru, 1991*, PNUD, Lima, July 1992.

Prontuario de Legislación Sanitaria del Perú, 4 vols, Imp. Americana, Lima, 1937.

Puglielli, L., Cattrini, C., Garces Resa, J.J, Velasques, L.M. and Garcia, León, 'Symptomless carriage of *Vibrio Cholera* in Peru', *Lancet*, **339**, 25 April 1992, 1056–7.

Pulgar Vidal, Javier, *Geografía del Perú, las ocho regiones naturales*, Peisa, Lima, 1987.

Quick, Robert E., Vargas, Rodolfo, Moreno, Dafne, Mujica, Oscar, Beingolea, Luis, Palacios, Ana María, Seminario, Luis and Tauxe, Robert V., 'Epidemic Cholera in the Amazon: The Challenge of Preventing Death', *American Journal of Tropical Medicine and Hygiene*, **48**, 5, 1993, 597–602.

Quirós, Manuel, 'Demostración de la vía que ha seguido la fiebre amarilla al invadir el norte del Perú', *La Crónica Médica*, **38**, 1921, 400.

Ramos Díaz, Arquímedes, 'Epidemiología de la peste bubónica en la sierra del departamento de Lambayeque', *Boletín de la Oficina Sanitaria Panamericana*, **17**, 1938, 776–81.

Ranger, Terence, and Slack, Paul, *Epidemics and Ideas, Essays on the History of Pestilence*, Cambridge University Press, Cambridge, 1992.

Rebagliati, Raúl, 'La situación epidemiológica del Perú en 1939', *Boletín de la Dirección de Salubridad Pública*, 1940, 240–65, Imp. Americana, Lima, 1940.

Registro Oficial de Fomento, Dirección de Salubridad Pública, La Opinión Nacional, Lima, 1905.

Reglamento del Servicio de vacunación y revacunación antivariólicas, Tipografía Lucero, Lima, 1908.

'Relación nominal de los señores médicos-cirujanos conforme al censo practicado de 1940', *Boletín de la Dirección de Salubridad Pública*, 1940, 180–89, Imp. Americana, Lima, 1940, 184.

Reyna, Carlos and Zapata, Antonio, *Crónica sobre el cólera en el Perú*, Desco, Lima, 1991.

Ribeyro, Julio E., *Saneamiento de Lima*, Imp. Gil, Lima, 1935.

Rico-Avelló, Carlos, *Historia de la Sanidad Española (1900–1925)*, Jimenez, S.A., Madrid, 1969.

Ries, Allen A., Vugia, Duc J., Beingolea, Luis, Palacios, Ana María, Vasquez, Esther, Wells, Joy G., García, Noe, Swerdlow, David L., Pollack, Marjorie, Bean, Nancy H., Seminarío, Luis and Tauxe, Robert V., 'Cholera in Piura, Peru: A Modern Urban Epidemic', *Journal of Infectious Diseases*, **166**, 6, 1992, 1429–33.

Risse, Guenter B., 'Epidemics Before Aids: A New Research Program', in Victoria A. Harden, and Guenther B. Risse (eds), *Aids and the Historian*, 2–12, National Institute of Health Publication, Washington, DC, 1991.

Riva Aguero, José de la., 'El obispo Sarasola', *Mercurio Peruano*, **206**, 1944, 3–24.

Roca, Erasmo, *Por la clase indígena*, Impresiones y Publicidad, Lima, 1935.

Rodriguez, Marcela, Tejada, Edgar, Swerdlow, David L., Mintz, Eric D, Ocampo, Cecilia, Espejo, Luis, Saldaña, Wilton, Seminario, Luis, Pollack, Marjorie and Tauxe, Robert V., 'Epidemia de Cólera en el Distrito de Víctor Larco Herrera, Trujillo, La Libertad', *Revista Peruana de Epidemiología*, **4**, 2, 1991, 2–6.

Rodríguez Ocaña, Esteban (ed.), *La Constitución de la Medicina Social como disciplina en España (1822–1923)*, Ministerio de Sanidad, Madrid, 1987.

Romero, Emilio, *Monografía del Departamento de Puno*, Imp. Torres Aguirre, Lima, 1928.

Rosenberg, Charles, *The Cholera Years: The United States in 1832, 1849, and 1866*, University of Chicago Press, Chicago, 1962.

———, *Explaining Epidemics and Other Studies in the History of Medicine*, Cambridge University Press, Cambridge, 1992.

Ruxin, Joshua N., 'Magic Bullet: The History of Oral Rehydration Therapy', *Medical History*, **38**, 1991, 363–97.

Salud y los servicios básicos, Coordinadora de ONGs para el Cólera, Chimbote, 1993.

Sarasola, Sabas, 'Mensaje misionero', *Misiones Dominicanas del Perú*, **72**, 1932, 161–7.

———, 'Extraña epidemia en la región del Urubamba', *Misiones Dominicanas del Perú*, **74**, 1933, 2–9.

———, 'De Quillabamba: hacia la desolación', *Misiones Dominicanas del Perú*, **77**, 1933, 121–5.

———, 'El Proceso de la epidemia en la región del Urubamba', *Misiones Dominicanas del Perú*, **75**, 1933, 41–7.

———, 'Del Urubamba: el paludismo, hacia la normalidad', *Misiones Dominicanas del Perú*, **83**, 1934, 121–7.

Seminario, Luis, Lopez, Augusto, Vásquez, Esther and Rodríguez, Marcela, 'Epidemia del cólera en el Perú, vigilancia epidemiológica', *Revista Peruana de Epidemiología*, **4**, 2, 1991, 8–10.

El Servicio Cooperativo Interamericano de Salud Pública, 15 años de actividad, Embajada de Estados Unidos en Perú, Lima, 1958.

Servicio Especial de Salud Pública, *Informe Anual de actividades*, SESP, Lima, 1965.

Servicio Nacional Antimalárico, 'Hacia la antarquía en el control de la malaria en el Peru', in *Primeras Jornadas Médico Quirurgicas del Norte del Perú*, Laboratorios ABEEFE, Tryillo, 1945.

———, *La Lucha Antimalárica en el Perú: Leyes, decretos y resoluciones*, Dirección de Salubridad Pública, Lima, 1945.

Servicio de Sanidad Militar, *Cartilla de propaganda antipalúdica*, Ministerio de Guerra, La Punta, 1928.

———, *Campaña contra el paludismo; instrucciones detalladas para la mejor aplicación del plan de lucha contra esta enfermedad*, Ministerio de Guerra, Lima, 1932.

———, 'Editorial, factores de cooperación en la conquista sanitaria de la selva', *Revista de Sanidad Militar*, **7**, 1934, 5–8.

Shannon, Raymond C., 'Observaciones sobre el *Anopheles Pseudopunctipennis* en el Perú', *Revista de la Sanidad Militar*, **3**, 1930, 11–33.

El siglo XX en el Perú a través de 'El Comercio' 1901–1910, El Comercio, Lima, 1991.

Silva, Renán, *Las Epidemias de la Viruela de 1782 y 1802 en la Nueva Granada*, Universidad del Valle, Cali, 1992.

'La situación del cólera en las Américas', *Boletín Epidemiológico, Organización Panamericana de la Salud*, **15**, 1, 1994, 13–16.

'Situación del cólera en las Américas, 1996', *Boletín Epidemiologico, Organización Panamericana de la Salud*, **18**, 1997, 7.

'Situación de salud en las Américas. Selección de inicadores básicos, 1996', *Boletín Epidemiológico, Organización Panamericana de la Salud*, **18**, 1997, 8–9.

Slack, Paul, *The Impact of Plague in Tudor and Stuart England*, Oxford University Press, Oxford, 1990.

Sneyder, J.D. and Blake, P.A., 'Is Cholera a Problem for U.S. Travelers?', *Journal of American Medical Association*, **247**, 1982, 2268–9.

'Sobre una encuesta iniciada para conocer la epidemiología nacional, Yungay', *Boletín de la Dirección de Salubridad Pública*, 1918, 346–53, La Opinión Nacional, Lima, 1918.

Stepan, Nancy, 'The Interplay between Socio-Economic Factors and Medical Science: Yellow Fever Research in Cuba and the United States', *Social Studies of Science*, **8**, 1978, 397–424.

Stiglich, Germán, *Geografía comentada del Perú*, Sanmarti, Lima, 1913.

Strode, George K. (ed.), *Yellow Fever*, McGraw-Hill, New York, 1951.

Suarez, Rubén and Bradford, Bonnie, *The Economic Impact of the Cholera Epidemic in Peru*, Environmental Health Project, Washington, DC, 1993.

Swerdlow, David L., Allen, M.D. and Ries, A., 'Cholera in the Americas, Guidelines for the Clinicia', *Journal of the American Medical Association*, **267**, 11, 1992, 1495–9.

Swerdlow, David L., Mintz, Eric D., Rodriguez, Marcela, Tejada, Edgar, Ocampo, Cecilia, Espejo, Luis, Greene, Katherine, Saldaña, Wilton, Seminario, Luis, Tauxe, Robert V., Wells, Joy G., Bean, Nancy H., Ries, Allen A., Pollack, Marjorie, Vertiz, B. and Blake, P., 'Waterborne Transmission of Epidemic Cholera in Trujillo, Peru: Lessons for a Continent at Risk', *Lancet*, **340**, 1992, 28–32.

Szymonski, Zszislaw, *Enfermedades Tropicales*, Azángaro, Lima, 1936.

Taller de Estudios, Fanny Abanto Calle, *Geografía de Cajamarca*, Labrusa, Cajamarca,1990.

Tamayo, Manuel and Mostajo, Benjamín, 'Cremación y utilización de la basuras de Lima', *La Crónica Médica*, **409**,1906, 1–6.

Tamayo Herrera, José, *Historia Social del Cuzco Republicano*, Industrial Gráfica, Lima, 1978.

———, *Historia social e indigenismo en el altiplano*, Ed. Treintaitres, Lima, 1982.

———, *Historia del Indigenismo Cuzqueño, siglos XVI–XX*, Instituto Nacional de Cultura, Lima, 1988.

Tauxe, Robert V. and Blake, Paul A., 'Letter from Peru, Epidemic Cholera in Latin America', *Journal of the American Medical Association*, **267**, 10, 1992, 1388–90.

Teel, Charles, 'Missionaries, Visionaries and Revolutionaries, Logging a Passage in Search of Fernando and Ana Stahl', *Adventist Heritage*, **12**, 1988, 3–14.

———, 'Las raíces radicales del adventismo en el altiplano peruano', *Allpanchis*, **33**, 1989, 209–48.

Temkin, Owsei, *Studies in Intellectual History*, Johns Hopkins University Press, Baltimore, MD, 1953.

Tocón, Carmen, and Acosta, Antonio, *Con la vida a cuestas, mujer, empleo y condiciones de vida*, Casa de la Mujer, Chimbote, 1994.

Torrealva, Félix, 'Algunas observaciones sobre el paludismo en Ica', *Revista de la Sanidad de la Policía*, **2**, 1942, 11–16.

Tulchin, Joseph S. and Baland, Gary (eds), *Peru in Crisis, Dictatorship or Democracy*, Woodrow Wilson Center, Washington, DC, 1994.

Ugarte, Luis and Geller, Samuel, 'La Opinión de los médicos sanitario departamental, y titular de La Convención', *La Reforma Médica*, **117**, 1933, 511–12.

Ugarte Ochoa, Marco Aurelio (ed.), *La Convención, el trabajo y sus luchas sociales*, Imp. Amauta, Cuzco, 1983.

Ureta del Solar, Alberto, 'El Saneamiento urbano en el Perú', *Boletín de la Escuela de Ingenieros del Perú*, **19**, 1946, 3–76.

Urrunaga, Roberto and Wicht, Juan Julio (eds), *Informe de coyuntura, evolución de la economía peruana, 1992, segundo semestre*, Universidad del Pacífico, Lima, 1993.

US Department of State, *Publication 2803: Health and Sanitation Program, Agreement between the United States of America and Peru*, Government Printing Office, Washington, DC, 1947.

———, *Publication 5400: Health and Sanitation Cooperative Program in Peru*, Government Printing Office, Washington, DC, 1955.

Valcárcel, Luis E., *Tempestad en los Andes*, Minerva, Lima, 1927.

———, *Memorias*, Instituto de Estudios Peruanos, Lima, 1981.

Valdizán, Hermilio, *Diccionario de medicina peruana*, 3 vols, Talleres Larco Herrera, Lima, 1923.

———, *Los Médicos italianos en el Perú*, Comité Pro-cociera italiana Nell' America Latina, Lima, 1924.

Valdizán, Hermilio and Maldonado, Angel, *La Medicina Popular Peruana (Contribución al Folklore Médico del Perú)*, 3 vols, Imp. Torres Aguirre, Lima, 1922.

Valencia, F., 'Aymachura y muru', *Archivos Peruanos de Folklore*, **2**, 1953, 87–90.

Vargas, M., Huicho, L., Salcedo, V. and Monge, E., 'The Use of Isotonic Sodium Chloride in the Early Treatment of Cholera Diarrhea: The Peruvian Experience', *Journal of Wilderness Medicine*, **4**, 1993, 62–7.

Vasques, Esther, Palacios, Ana María, Beingolea, Luis, Ries, Allen A., Vugia, Duc J., Wells, Joy G., Seminario, Luis, Pollack, Marjorie and Tauxe, Robert V., 'Epidemia de cólera en Perú: estudio caso-control de Piura', *Revista Peruana de Epidemiología*, **4**, 2, 1991, 47–50.

Vasquez Lapeyre, Luis, 'Patología y población indígena del Perú', *Perú Indígena*, **2**, 1952, 48–55.

Vidal, Carlos, 'El cólera en el Perú', *Revista Médica Herediana*, **2**, 1991, 52–3.

Villalobos, Enrique, 'Servicio Nacional Antimalárico', *Boletín de la Dirección de Salubridad Pública*, 1943, 25–30, Minerva, Lima, 1943.

Webb, Richard and Fernández Baca, Graciela, *Perú en números 1991, Anuario Estadístico*, Cuanto, Lima, 1991.

Webb, Sheila, *Waterborne Diseases in Perú*, The World Bank policy research working papers, Washington, DC, August 1992.

Weiss, Pedro, 'Geografía de las Enfermedades en el Perú en relación con las zonas climáticas', in *Conferencias de Ciencias Antropológicas, Actas, y Trabajos*, 140–67, Universidad de San Marcos, Lima, 1951.

———, *Geografía de las enfermedades en el Perú, fascículo costa*, Ed. San Marcos, Lima, 1955.

Weiss, Pedro, Rojas, Hector and Guzman Barrón, Alberto, *Informe presentado por la comisión organizada por la Dirección de Salubridad para estudiar la región del Madre de Dios*, Imp. Americana, Lima, 1924.

Westphal, Edward A., 'Servicio Cooperativo Interamericano de Salud Pública', *Boletín de la Dirección de Salubridad Pública*, 1943, 91–6, Minerva, Lima, 1944.

Westphal, Edward A. and Horton, Robert K., 'Malaria control in Chimbote, Peru', *Boletín de la Oficina Sanitaria Panamericana*, **25**, 1946, 796–809.

Williams, Greer, *Virus Hunters, The Lives and Triumphs of Great Modern Medical Pioneers*, Alfred A. Knopf, London, 1960.

Willie, Johanes, 'La Fauna anofelina malarígena de las zonas cálidas del Cuzco', *Revista Médica*, **196**, 1934, 645.

Wise, David O., 'Vanguardismo a 3,800 metros: el caso del *Boletín Titikaka* (Puno, 1926–1930)', *Fénix*, **30–31**, 1984, 257–69.

———, 'La Sierra (Lima, 1927–1930) La Voz de los Hombres del Ande.', *Fénix*, **34–5**, 1989, 70–105.

World Bank, *Peru, Lima Water Supply and Sewerage Project, Loan 2139-PE*, World Bank Report 10230, Washington, DC, 1991.

Zinsser, Hans, *Rats, Lice and History, the Biography of a Bacillus*, Little Brown and Co., Boston, 1934.

Zschock, Dieter K., *Health Care in Peru: Resources and Policy*, Westview Press, Boulder, CO, 1988.

Zulueta, J. de, 'Malaria and Ecosystems: From Prehistory to Posteradication', *Parrasitologia*, **36**, 1994, 7–15.

Unpublished sources

Alván, José R., 'La fiebre amarilla en Tamarindo y Catacaos', Bachelor thesis, Universidad Nacional Mayor de San Marcos, 1920.

Amorín, Luis, 'Mi experiencia personal en la campaña contra la Peste', Bachelor thesis, Universidad Nacional Mayor de San Marcos, 1930.

Aragón, Carlos, 'La malaria en los valles de La Convención y Lares, sector Echerate, 1936–1939', Bachelor thesis, Universidad Nacional Mayor de San Marcos, 1941.

Bensimón, Amalia and Diaz, Graciela, 'Factores que influyen en la incidencia de las Enfermedades Diarréicas Agudas (EDA) en niños menores de 1 año, Iquitos', Licenciate thesis, Universidad Nacional de la Amazonía Peruana, 1991.

Boza, Julio, 'Contribución al estudio de la peste bubónica', Bachelor thesis, Universidad Nacional Mayor de San Marcos, 1916.

Buroncle Diaz, Carlos G., 'Vacunación contra la viruela en el Perú en los últimos 20 años', Bachelor thesis, Universidad Nacional Mayor de San Marcos, 1970.

Cortez, Miguel, 'Epidemia palúdica de los valles de la Convención y Lares', Bachelor thesis, Universidad Nacional Mayor de San Marcos, 1938.

Cruz, Porfirio S. de la, 'Aspectos epidemiológicos actuales de la malaria en el Perú. Control y trabajos iniciales de erradicación', Bachelor thesis, Universidad Nacional Mayor de San Marcos, 1954.

Cuzquen, Leopoldo, 'Epidemiología de la malaria en el Perú', PhD thesis, Universidad Nacional Mayor de San Marcos, 1976.

Donayre, R., 'Contribuciónal estudio entomológico de la malaria en el Perú, departamiento del Cuzco, valle de La Convención', Bachelor thesis, Universidad Nacional Mayor de San Marcos, 1947.

Gálvez, Carmela and Regalado, Dianera, 'Efectividad de 4 plantas de uso tradicional en el tratamiento de enfermedades parasitarias gastrointestinales de 1–5 años, Cajamarca, 1991', Licenciate thesis, Universidad Nacional de Cajamarca, 1991.

Heredia, César, 'Endemoepidemiología de una enfermedad evanescente', Bachelor thesis, Universidad Nacional Mayor de San Marcos, 1960.

Iturri, José Antonio, 'A epidemia de cólera no Peru como um evento social. As representacoes das liderancas comunitárias de Villa El Salvador, Lima 1991', Master thesis, School of Public Health, Fundación Oswaldo Cruz, 1994.

Luglio, J. Mario, 'Campaña antimalárica en La Convención y Yanatile', Bachelor thesis, Universidad Nacional Mayor de San Marcos, 1950.

Macedo, Flora and Ríos, Susana, 'Efectividad de la terapia de rehidratación oral, Hospital Iquitos', Licenciate thesis, Universidad Nacional de la Amazonía Peruana, 1985.

Maltby, Laura L., 'Indian Revolts in the Altiplano and the Conquest of the Land, 1895–1925', Bachelor thesis, Harvard University, 1972.

McNulty, Luis, 'Contribución al estudio de la peste en el Perú', Bachelor thesis, Universidad Nacional Mayor de San Marcos, 1912.

Odicio, Aníbal, 'Contribución a la seroterapia de la peste', Bachelor thesis, Universidad Nacional Mayor de San Marcos, 1911.

Ortega, Segundo, 'La peste en el Perú, desde su aparición hasta 1924', Bachelor thesis, Universidad Nacional Mayor de San Marcos, 1925.

Perez, Víctor, 'Algunas consideraciones relativas a la etiología, patogenia, tratamiento y profilaxia de la peste en Lima', Bachelor thesis, Universidad Nacional Mayor de San Marcos, 1923.

Portella, Juan A., 'La higiene en las casas de vecindad, necesidad de construir casas higiénicas para obreros', Bachelor thesis, Universidad Nacional Mayor de San Marcos, 1903.

Ríos Dávila, Javier, 'Impacto de la epidemia del cólera y la huelga de salud en el servicio de emergencia, 1991', Medical thesis, Universidad Peruana Cayetano Heredia, 1993.

Rosales, Amador, 'Algunas consideraciones profilácticas observadas en la epidemia de fiebre amarilla en Paiján', Bachelor thesis, Universidad Nacional Mayor de San Marcos, 1924

Sanchez, Andrea, Vargas, Olga and Villacorta, Isolina, 'Actitud de la población en la no utilización del servicio de salud, Llacanora, Cajamarca', Licenciate thesis, Universidad Nacional de Cajamarca, 1987.

Urteaga, Luis C., 'Estudio clínico y epidemiológico del cólera, Hospital Regional Guzmán Barrón, Chimbote, 1991', Master thesis, Universidad Peruana Cayetano Heredia, 1994.

Vargas, Javier, 'Diarrea aguda y estado nutricional en niños menores de 5 años atendidos en el Hospital Regional del Amazonas', Medical thesis, Universidad Nacional de la Amazonía Peruana, 1993.

Zapata, Carlos E., 'La fiebre amarilla en Piura', Bachelor thesis, Universidad Nacional Mayor de San Marcos, 1920.

Index